DR. SEBI CURE FOR HERPES

Discover the Proven 3-Step Method That Allowed 7000+ People to Get Rid Forever of Cold Sores and Genital Herpes With No Medication

By Serena Brown

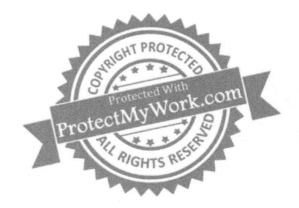

Table of Contents

A FREE BOOK FOR YOU! (<u>DOWNLOAD IT</u>)

- Are you interested in **getting rid of toxins** and nourishing your body?
- Are you curious about how Dr. Sebi used to **face disease and strengthen the immune system**?

Introducing...

"*DR. SEBI: 7-Day Full-Body Detox for Beginners*" → **100% FREE FOR YOU!**

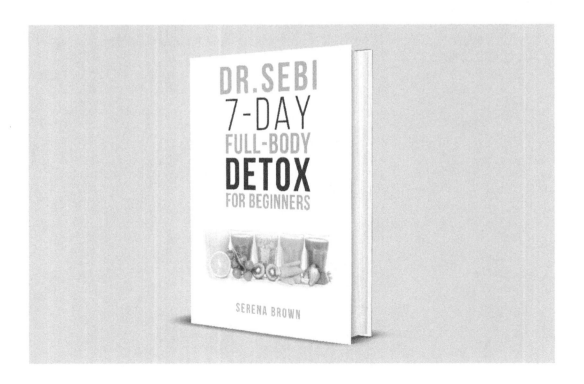

SCAN THE QR CODE BELOW TO DOWNLOAD IT FOR FREE!!!

Chapter 1: Herpes Simplex Virus

What's Herpes?

It is indeed a virus that might stay inactive or allow the body to undergo the flare-up. Two major strains are known.

While the herpes virus group has eight variants, including the Epstein-Barr virus, we will concentrate on the two most prevalent HSV types.

HSV-1, or oral herpes, is a type of herpes spread by saliva. Many persons with oral herpes were possibly compromised during infancy or adulthood by exchanging a straw, cup, eating utensils, toothbrush, gum, or kissing.

Among the most prevalent sexual diseases is HSV-2, also identified as genital herpes. The incidents involving genital herpes within that U.S. are above 1 in 6 people aged 14-49, as per the C.D.C. In women, it is often around twice as high as in males.

Herpes infection is drawn-out contamination that is brought about by the herpes simplex virus (HSV). The genital district, the oral locale, the skin, and the butt-centric area are the body areas influenced by this infection.

This ailment is known for an extremely prolonged period, and it normally assaults people causing a few ailments; some are mellow, and some are perilous.

Genital herpes is one of the most widely recognized kinds of herpes simplex infection. The genital herpes infection is an explicitly transmitted disease that affects to genital and butt-centric rankles. There might be bruises which additionally influence the mouth and face.

A few instances of the rehashed appearance of genital herpes are brought about by H.V.S. 2. A large portion of this disease is spread from victims who don't realize they have it, and more often than not, the side effects are asymptomatic in a victim.

People can contract this contamination through a sexual relationship with a victim infected with HSV. Additionally, you can get contaminated by your sex accomplice who doesn't encounter any indications of this disease whatsoever.

More so, the subsequent kind can be brought about by oral-butt-centric contact or butt-centric contact with a victim. HSV 2 is the most predominant herpes infection disease, yet the HSV 1 happens less ordinarily.

HSV-1

The primary way that the HSV-1 virus spreads is through an outbreak from an affected person. In America alone, it is estimated that 67% of people under the age of 49 are infected with the HSV-1 herpes virus. But most of these people may not experience an outbreak throughout their lifetime.

The Ways You Can Contact the Herpes Simplex Virus

The ways you can contact HSV-1 includes:

- Kissing someone infected.

- Making use of the same eating utensils that an already affected person is making use of.

- Using the same lipstick or lip balm with an affected person.

- Engaging in oral sex with an infected person.

HSV-2

The primary way to contact HSV-2 is through sexual contact with an already affected person. According to the American Academy of Dermatology (A.A.D.), 20 to 25% of active sexually are already infected with the HSV-2 herpes virus.

This one is not that common like the type one as only 15.5% of people from the age of 14—49 are suffering from this type of herpes in the U.S.A.

It is 100% impossible for you to get infected with genital herpes through a toilet seat.

You can also get infected through oral sex.

Different Manifestation of the Herpes Virus

Cold Sore

We'll expose many herpes myths in this book, but here's one of the most prevalent; the idea that a "cold sore" is NOT herpes. A lot of people believe this because of the way the virus is marketed.

Knowledge about herpes is mostly the result of marketing firms tinkering with public perception.

However, not all mouth sorer is related to the herpes virus.. A dermatologist can identify herpes sore versus a different type of mouth ulcer.

Herpes Zoster

Herpes zoster is the clinical manifestation of the reactivation of the Varicella Zoster virus (VZV), the primary infection of chickenpox, an exanthemata's disease affecting mainly children and characterized by maculae, bumps, blisters (vesicles), and crusts.

The viral D.N.A. finds shelter in the posterior sensory ganglia or the cranial pars. Different factors comprising stress, immune depression, lymphomas, or immunosuppressive drugs may trigger this genetic material's activation and progress towards the epidermis. This triggering effect can take place at any time. However, it prevails in people who are older or have a depressed immune system. It is not season-related.

The VZV belongs to the Herpes virus family and comprises a double-chain D.N.A. genome with a lipoprotein layer that helps the virus adhere and get into.

It gains access through the airway and replicates in the rachidian nerves' ganglia, resulting in the first viridian.

Chickenpox

The virus gains access through the respiratory epithelium and replicates in the lymph nodes, spreading through the blood and resulting in chickenpox. Symptoms do not take more than 15 days. The virus remains inside the posterior lymph nodes.

It starts as a hyperesthetic, painful, prodigious area preceded by fever, cephalea, asthenia, and local discomfort. Then, small blisters appear erythematous, the well-delimited place that adopts a radicular distribution. These blisters, which completely cover the area, tend to meet and group into a single one. Scorching, neritic pain is characteristic and can persist for months (post-herpetic neuralgia).

Pyogenic impetiginization is frequent at the level of the skin, and mucopurulent conjunctivitis in the ophthalmic region. It can mainly be seen in older people. It can be continuous or parodist. There is also paralysis, esp. in the face and the lumbosacral region and paresis. Despite its low incidence, encephalitis can also be a complication, presenting with fever, meningeal signs, disturbance of consciousness, hallucinations, and delirium.

What Are the Causes of Herpes?

There are some primary causes of herpes, which I am going to talk about below:

Oral sex

Oral sex is good, and I do not deny it, but it is wise for us to know who and how healthy our partner's mouth is. If the mouth of the person giving you a leader has cold sores around his/her mouth, there is a tendency that you might get infected with herpes.

Unprotected sex

Having unprotected sex with someone suffering from herpes transmits the virus.

Sharing sex toys with someone infected with the herpes virus transmits the virus rapidly and very fast.

Transmitted through birth

Another craziest thing about this virus is that it can be transmitted from the mother to her newborn baby through birth delivery if the mother's genital herpes have sores while giving birth.

Please note that the sharing of towels, chairs, kitchen utensils, or toilet seats with someone with herpes cannot get you infected because the viruses need a moist environment to be transmitted. That is why it can be transmitted through the eyes, anus, vagina, mouth, and wounds.

The Symptoms of the Herpes Virus Include

The main symptoms of the herpes virus are something that everyone needs to recognize to be careful because a lot of people with the herpes virus show no symptoms or visible signs such:

Urine and Discharge Problems for Women

At the point when pee comes into contact with an open injury, stinging is a typical sensation. Ladies experience more difficulty with pee ignoring the wounds than men due to the shape and position of the urethra. Ladies may likewise observe a release adjustment when the herpes infection is dynamic. Rather than white, watery, and normally unscented, the release might be thick, with a yellow tinge and a sharp smell. This is an indication of disease in the cervix.

Blisters inside the Urethra

The urethra is the cylinder that interfaces the urinary bladder to the private parts. In the two people with herpes type-2, difficult bruises can frame on this cylinder's inward coating. While peeing, an individual may feel a consuming or extremely sharp steel sensation when pee disregards these bruises. Not at all like genital or mouth bruises, the specialist may need to lead tests to affirm a herpes disease when the urethra is influenced.

Fatigue

Individuals with a herpes infection contamination may see general sentiments of tiredness and shortcoming and an absence of vitality. Weakness may likewise discover its way into the muscles, leaving them feeling agonizing or substantial. This side effect can likewise cause brevity of breath, weight reduction, uneasiness, and gloom, and leave individuals feeling like they have to nap as often as possible during the day.

Spinal pains

The herpes type-2 infection can influence the lumbar and sacral nerve roots, prompting nerve and nerve endings issues. Individuals with a herpes viral contamination can create torment in the lower back, posterior, and thighs, particularly if the disease is revolved around the privates. This sort is regularly intermittent and can be very awkward and excruciating.

Flu-Like Symptoms

Influenza-like side effects that can create alongside a herpes contamination include a fever with cools, an irritated throat, diligent hack, and a runny or stuffy nose. A few people may encounter sickness and retching or the runs. The safe framework kicks vigorously to battle the contamination, yet until it can finish its work, the herpes infection leaves many people feeling exhausted.

Headaches

Headaches and the herpes infection go connected at the hip when a flare-up happens. Indications of headaches incorporate general head torment, which can move from a moderate, dull yearn to an extreme, throbbing agony behind the eyes. Different side effects incorporate peevishness and affectability to sound and light. This cerebral pain may cause summed up muscle throbs, inconvenience dozing or focusing, obscured vision, nausea, and craving loss.

Swollen Lymph Nodes

Lymph hubs are little bean-formed organs all through the body. The lymphatic framework goes about as a seepage or sifting activity, conveying lymph liquid, supplements, and waste material through the tissues and the circulation system. Generally found in the neck, the crotch, and under the arms, these hubs expand and become delicate during disease or damage. When somebody has genital herpes, the organs around the genital territory will expand and might be sore.

Blisters on the Genitals

When genital rankles, happen, the herpes type-2 infection (HSV 2) is as often as possible suspected as a reason. It will initially begin with a comparative inclination to that of the mouth wounds, yet with greater power because of the zone's affectability.

Around 12 to 24 hours before noticeable rankles, the skin will be bothersome and excruciating and might be red, crude, and broke. At that point, a rankle will show up burst open to turn into an ulcer before scabbing over to mend. The herpes episodes can repeatedly happen; however, the manifestations of bunched rankles will here and there become less extreme than the underlying disease. The infection is infectious both during an episode and when there are no manifestations or wounds.

Mouth blisters

As often as possible, mouth blisters on the mouth brought about by the herpes type-1 infection (HSV-1) are a typical event. After they initially create individuals powerless to them contract the bruises over and over. Most normally found around the lips, the herpes infection can likewise cause rankles in the mouth and throat.

The mouth blisters start as little red fixes that transform into a rankle or a bunch of rankles that blast and leave a crude, sobbing region in the long run blast. This territory normally recuperates and scabs over without assistance, yet over-the-counter creams can help alleviate and fix the skin.

Itching or Tingling Around Genitals or Anus

The main indication of the herpes infection flare-up is tingling and bothering around the influenced zone. The tainted individual may feel a shivering or tingling sensation around the private parts of the butt or some other delicate tissue territory like the mouth or nose. This is an indication that will create in this limited territory. The skin will get red, irritated, and may break a bit. It will feel crude and sore, and contacting is prompted against as this can move germs and microorganisms.

What Triggers Herpes?

Through skin-to-skin touch with anyone who got the infection, herpes can quickly be transmitted. You will get it, typically through anal, oral, & vaginal intercourse, anytime your mouth or genitals meet their mouth and genitals.

If there's a path for herpes to get through, such as a wound, rash, burn, or other infections, other skin areas may get contaminated. To get herpes, you may not have to have intercourse. Herpes may also be spread in non-sexual contexts, such as whether you are pecked on the lips by a parent with a cold sore. While they were children, most individuals having oral herpes developed it. While vaginal childbirth, a mother may transfer herpes to the new-born, but that's very uncommon.

If you tap herpes sore and touch your genitals, eyes, or mouth without washing the hands first, you will transmit herpes to any other areas of your body. This way, you will even move herpes onto somebody else.

Herpes is more common when the sores are exposed and moist since the infection is quickly transmitted by fluid through herpes blisters. Although there have been no sores, herpes may still "shed" & get passed on to someone, and the skin appears perfectly fine.

The majority of people receive herpes through someone who has no sores at all. It will remain in the body for a long time without showing some signs, but it is impossible to tell for certain how and where you caught it. That's why it's a pretty sly virus that so many individuals have herpes.

You can't catch herpes by hugging, shaking hands, sneezing, coughing, or using toilet seats because the infection dies rapidly outside of the body.

The individual must refrain from oral, anal, or vaginal sex with someone affected with HSV-2 to avoid contractions with genital herpes. To do this, you should refrain from sex entirely or just have sex in a legally monogamous partnership in which neither spouse exhibits genital herpes.

The use of contraceptives might even minimize the risk of genital herpes, but lesions could be present in places that are not covered by condoms, and no lesions need to be visible for the disease to spread. Some strategies to avoid or minimize the transmission of the infection can involve taking medicine each day to avoid an epidemic, or after an epidemic, avoiding participating in anal, oral, or vaginal intercourse.

The factors that can trigger an outbreak of the herpes virus include:

- Prolonged stress or stressful activities

- Excessive heat or sunburn

- Fever

- Menstruation

Manifestations of Herpes Virus

1. ## It happens through the change of existing infections

In general, R.N.A. infections will have an uncommonly high pace of change since mistakes in recreating their R.N.A. genomes are not rectified by editing. Some transformation changes their current infections into new hereditary assortments that can cause illness, even resistance to the infection.

2. ## Distribution of herpes infection from a little secluded human populace

For example, aids went un-named and unnoticed for a considerable length of time before it started to spread the world over. Accordingly, mechanical and social elements, including reasonable worldwide travel, blood transfusions, extramarital perversion, and the maltreatment of intravenous medications, permitted a formerly uncommon human illness to turn into a worldwide one.

3. ## The spread of existing infection from different creatures

Researchers evaluated that seventy-five percent of new human infections start along these lines. Creatures hold and transmit a specific infection; however, they are commonly unaffected by it are said to go about as a characteristic supply for that infection (Campbell Reece, 2008).

The Risk of Contracting the Herpes Virus

Everyone can contract the herpes virus, but certain factors expose some people to the risk of contracting the herpes virus.

Some of such risk factors include:

- Having a weak immune system

- Having oral and unprotected sex with affected partners

- Having a previously untreated sexually transmitted disease

- Having multiple sexual partners at a young age

- More risk as a woman

Who's at risk of getting diseases of herpes simplex?

Anyone, irrespective of age, maybe contaminated by HSV. Almost exclusively, the probability is dependent on susceptibility to the virus.

Individuals are increasingly at risk in sexual transmission instances because they have intercourse that is not covered by contraceptives or other protective techniques.

Some HSV-2 risk factors include: • Having several sex partners • Physical intercourse at an earlier age • Female being • Getting another virus spread via sex • Possession of a compromised immune system When a pregnant lady has a genital herpes infection at the period of delivery, the infant will be subjected to both forms of HSV and will be at risk of severe complications.

What is the future regarding herpes simplex in the long-term?

For the remainder of their life, individuals who get contaminated from HSV may have the infection. The infection can continue to exist in an infected individual's nerve cells, although it doesn't show symptoms.

Frequent outbreaks can occur in certain persons. After they have become bitten, some can only undergo one infection, and afterward, the virus might be inactive.

Over time, it is suspected that occurrence -become less frequent when the body continues to produce antibodies. There are normally no risks if a typically stable individual is afflicted with infection.

Preventing the transmission of diseases with herpes simplex

While there is no treatment for herpes, you should take precautions to discourage or avoid the spread of HSV to some other person from transmitting the virus.

If you have an HSV-1 epidemic, try taking just a few protective steps:

• Try preventing overt physical interaction with many other persons.

• Don't exchange certain things such as towels, cups, clothes, silverware, lip balm, or makeup, which can transmit the virus out.

• In an occurrence, do not partake in sexual contact, kissing, or some such form of sexual interaction.

• To avoid contact with lesions, clean your hands well & use medicine using cotton swabs.

Individuals with HSV-2 can prevent some form of sexual contact with the other persons. A contraceptive must be used through sex if the individual is not having signs but has also been confirmed having the virus. However, the infection may also be transmitted from exposed skin to a mate, including while using the contraceptive.

To keep the pathogen from harming their new-born infants, people who are expecting & contaminated might just have to use medication.

Chapter 2: Genital Herpes

Anyone sexually active can be infected with herpes. Herpes is a sexually transmitted disease caused by the herpes simplex virus. One can live with the virus without any symptoms, and that's the major reason it's easily spread through sexual intercourse. You can have the virus and spread it to your partner without knowing.

Generally, there are two types of viruses responsible for herpes infection. These viruses are; type 1 herpes simplex virus (HSV-1) and type 2 herpes simplex virus (HSV-2).

It's important to know that herpes doesn't only attack the genitals. Its infection can be oral. Oral herpes is mostly caused by herpes simplex virus type 1, which has a fever, blisters, cold sore, etc. However, in some cases, there may be no symptoms of the virus until its outbreak. It can be transmitted through saliva or oral sex.

Genital Herpes

Genital herpes is very common in the United States that one in every six persons has the virus. This so because it can easily be spread through sex. And one can easily be infected once he or she comes in contact with the virus. Using protection during sex is not a guarantee that the virus will not be transmitted.

If your skin touches your partner's infected area, whether genital or oral, you can be easily infected. With oral infection, the saliva of the infected person alone is enough to spread the disease. General secretions of someone infected with genital herpes can spread the disease.

So, herpes is a disease that can be spread, even without explicit sex. If you have oral sex with someone infected with oral herpes, you can get infected easily.

Though herpes can be spread easily through contact, the virus doesn't survive easily outside the body. You cannot contract the disease from objects like toilet seats, swimming pools, soap, towels, etc.

The best way to avoid herpes and other sexually transmitted diseases (S.T.D.s) is to avoid sex. However, if you are in a relationship, do your best to stick with your partner. Discuss with your couple if you notice any signs or symptoms of herpes. It's better to avoid sex if you have S.T.D.

Genital herpes is one of the most common sexually transmitted diseases in America; a clear understanding of this condition allows us to take appropriate measures to prevent it or even treat it if we have already acquired the disease.

Genital herpes is caused by the herpes simplex virus, which is estimated to be present in the body of one in five adults in the United States. Many people have no symptoms; therefore, they have no idea that they are infected with the virus.

After acquiring the disease, a lot of victims have recurrent episodes of genital ulcers for years. Genital infection can be managed with proper self-care and medication.

People with genital herpes are generally encouraged to discuss with the sexual partner, use condoms while having sex, and practice other preventive measures to prevent transmission to others. Genital herpes is transmittable even when there are no visible signs of ulcers and blisters.

Genital herpes is an infection that occurs near or on the genital. The type 2 herpes virus usually causes it. On the flip side, in recent years, the type 1 herpes infection is becoming more and more popular due to increased oral sex practice.

Contrary to some popular belief, skin contact is the only way to spread genital herpes. It can't be gotten through the sharing of towels, toilet seats, or swimming pools.

A significant outbreak is usually more severe than the subsequent ones. When the initial attack is over, it becomes inactive and does not cause symptoms again. This period is known as the dormant infection; any point after this, the herpes virus can pop up again. It then becomes reactive and once again causes sores.

Once a victim has contracted herpes, it is said to be there for life (which isn't true), and the person may experience repeated recurrences or outbreaks. Every single person has his/her unique recurrent pattern while experiencing episodes.

The frequency, severity, and duration of outbreaks can significantly be reduced with herbal treatments and mixtures.

What's the distinction between oral herpes & genital herpes?

Many people are uncertain about what to name these diseases, and that there occur two distinct forms of herpes viruses, which are HSV-1 & HSV-2, that may exist on multiple body sections. But it's pretty easy actually: It's labeled genital herpes anytime you either have HSV-1 or two on or near your vulva, vagina, butt, cervix, scrotum, penis, anus, inner thighs).

It's labeled oral herpes anytime you either have HSV-1 or 2 in or near your mouth, lips & throat. Fever blisters or Cold sores are often called oral herpes.

HSV-1 tends to cause oral herpes, & genital herpes is typically induced by HSV-2, with each strain choosing to reside in its favorite location. But with all forms of herpes, able to infect a region is entirely probable. For starters, when somebody having a cold sore over their lips offers you oral sex, you might develop HSV-1 over your genitals. And when you provide oral sex, someone having HSV-2 over their genitals, you will develop HSV-2 on the mouth.

Herpes and H.I.V.

Herpes sore on the skin, vagina, mouth, or rectum can provide a pathway for H.I.V. to easily enter the body. Moreover, genital herpes increase CD4 cells count in the lining of the genitals. CD4 cells are what H.I.V. usually targets to gain entry into the body.

When H.I.V. and Herpes are present in a person, they can easily spread the viruses during sexual intercourse.

Chapter 3: Herpes and Relationships

Telling Your Partner About HSV

So, now you're in the awkward position of having to explain to your significant other about being infected with genital herpes. Mainstream advice says: "tell your partner right away, always use condoms and take antiviral medication to lessen your partner's chance of contracting the disease."

What this common advice does not mention is the fact most people are terrified of HSV, and it's not uncommon, at all, for boyfriends and girlfriends to leave their partners over such a matter. It is not an easy subject to bring up!

Also, there's no mention of the severe side-effects of antiviral, and some doctors suggest taking them for the rest of your life to keep your partner from becoming infected!

While yes, obviously you need to tell your partner right away, I suggest approaching the topic from a slightly different frame of mind:

1. Explain You Have Hsv-2 Not "Genital Herpes"

Hysteria and taboos sometimes surround words and concepts more than anything else. Call the virus what it is. One of the reasons genital herpes is a bit of a misnomer is because sometimes HSV-2 isn't even located on the genitals, so if you're diagnosed with it, consult with your doctor to see if it's even latent on your nether region or not.

2. Explain the Virus Is Dormant and Prove It with a Medical Test

Prove your low viral count and static nature of the illness by having a urine test.

Explain the truth that catching HSV-2 is not a big deal, unlike what media/society/commercials say. Furthermore, provide some of the pamphlets provided by the herpes virus association.

Explain That You Take Natural Anti-Virals and You Lead a Lifestyle to Minimize Chances of Spreading It

Don't take dangerous antiviral pharmaceuticals if you're not having reoccurring outbreaks, and you don't need it. But reassure your partner that you're taking all the necessary precautions to prevent infecting anybody else.

Ask Him/Her If They've Ever Had a Cold Sore Before

If so, they are infected with HSV-1, a far more dangerous form of herpes. Explain 30-40% of the adult population also has HSV-2, and the number is growing.

Should I Tell My Partner About It?

It is a moral question, for which the answer is obviously "yes", but I can perfectly understand why many people debate the idea. Given the extreme social taboo of the virus, we've almost reached a point where people have no choice but to hide the fact they're infected, and I don't blame them. I don't condone it, but I perfectly understand why people feel this way.

It comes down to you; you can either be honest about your illness and risk having your partner leave you or be a liar and hide it. If it becomes apparent later that you're infected (or if he/she catches it from you), you'll risk having your partner leave you, and you'll be called a liar.

However, the big problem with revealing to a partner about herpes infection is that it's not realistic at the beginning of a relationship to wear the disease around your neck as a badge of dishonor. If you're single, and you meet the future love of your life, and you guys are tearing each other's clothes off in the heat of passion, do you think this is a good time to say, "wait, baby, I'm infected with genital herpes!"

Seriously, you'll never date again. Until the social taboo of HSV-2 is lifted, this will remain a big issue for everybody infected (which is currently 60+ million Americans).

For this reason, if you opt not to disclose herpes, make sure your viral count is as low as it can go, and wear a condom for added protection. The odds of a new partner contracting herpes, in this case, is very small.

If you're having any kind of outbreak whatsoever, you have to refrain from sex. Furthermore, if you're entering a relationship or a reoccurring series of physical encounters, reread the above steps for explaining your infection properly so as not to harm your relationship.

Dealing with the Herpes Stigma

The reason herpes is "the world's most annoying virus" is not so much because of the outbreaks as it is the social stigma associated with having it.

Herpes is considered a social taboo. It's used as an insult against people, and it's used by people who probably have HSV-2 without realizing it to denigrate others.

Which is a shame considering it's one of the most benign illnesses. HSV-1 does have some dangerous health ramifications, but HSV-2 (genital herpes) does not—unless you have an autoimmune disorder like H.I.V.

So why would anybody make something seem worse than it is? The answer is profit.

Because it's such a common illness, by scaring or shaming the people who catch it, it's possible to up the sales of Valtrex or whatever the latest pharmaceutical is. That's tens of millions of potential customers.

That is why many doctors indirectly exaggerate HSV in the media or on commercials. You'll never hear them say, "if you're one of the 2-4% who develops chronic HSV symptoms..." As far as they're concerned, everybody who is infected needs immediate pharmaceutical treatment.

Chapter 4: Dr. Sebi Thoughts on Herpes

An alkaline-rich diet rich in essential nutrients will help rid your body of the herpes virus. It can be achieved by creating an environment that can't support the growth of diseases causing substances.

The cells in your body require oxygen to perform to their optimum capacity, but the chemicals and substances found in some medicines and foods rob your cells the much-needed oxygen to thrive.

Curing the herpes virus requires adequate cleansing of your body, and Dr. Sebi's plant-based alkaline diet does just that.

It is essential to know that curing herpes depends on the types of food you eat and what you feed your body.

You should avoid eating sweets and starchy foods. Eat foods that are bitter instead of sweet.

Eat more healthy vegetables such as zucchini, mushrooms, squash, cactus leaf or cactus plant flowers, and sea vegetables. Plant-based iron, such as dandelion, burdock, and yellow dock, is also very helpful.

Dr. Sebi also emphasizes to practice fasting because fasting helps you to eat less and heal fast. Another good reason why Dr. Sebi's diet can cure herpes is that it eliminates mucus in your body. That is because once your mucus membrane is compromised, your immune system becomes weak, and you become to disease.

Your mucus membrane needs to remain healthy for you to be healthy because it is your mucus membrane in charge of protecting your body's cells.

The plant-based diets and herbs that are the main constituents of Dr. Sebi's alkaline cell foods are very effective for curing herpes.

Dr. Sebi was able to cure herpes by detoxifying the body and effectively nourishing the body.

You presumably know at this point what Dr. Sebi herpes fix is. Truly, Dr. Sebi's solution for herpes is continuously arriving at each side of the world. The purpose of it picking up prevalence so brisk isn't many dollars spent on commercials. Nor is it well known because some big-name is embracing it. It is dazzling the hearts of herpes patients in such a case that its adequacy.

Basic because the recuperating standards of this incredible cultivator are successful, the present reality is discussing him. Everybody today knows him as a man who helped millions conquer the illnesses wherein allopathy helped less. Notwithstanding, later on, it was understood that Dr. Sebi's standards were extraordinary in all the wellbeing inconveniences. Today, we won't just discuss what Dr. Sebi's herpes fix is about, yet we will reveal to you why Dr. Sebi's herpes fix is the best alternative you ought to go for.

Dr. Sebi was a famous herbalist who mended numerous patients when allopathic specialists couldn't give any assistance. He identified the enchantment that herbs conveyed and utilizing that supernatural made numerous lives excellent and sickness free. Similar standards of mending, when applied to herpes, gave sudden and incomprehensible outcomes. What the allopathic specialists couldn't reply, what the researchers couldn't stop can be fixed with the assistance of Dr. Sebi's remedy for herpes.

Nothing was taking a shot at mouth blisters and different manifestations of herpes. Yet, this botanist had at the top of the priority list some marvel herbs that can give another opportunity for herpes patients to live.

Even though it is likewise critical to perceive how it is done, at the same time, before that, let us see why Dr. Sebi's method is the best accessible option for you.

1. *It is the best because it works in herpes:* This is the best treatment so far from the effectiveness point of view. There is very little effective herpes treatment around the globe. There are antiviral drugs that are expensive but ineffective. They only give you a fake feeling of wellness when, in fact, nothing is working as it should in your body. Despite the intake of antiviral drugs by some herpes patients, the herpes simplex virus still thrives without limitation. It is a lot of sacrifices to choose antiviral drugs over traditional medicines as the former only pamper the symptoms of herpes with many underlying side effects. Some other herbs are safe but do not produce the same effect as Dr. Sebi's cure. It makes Dr.

Sebi's treatment the only solution that is perfect for every herpes patient as nothing comes close to its healing prowess.

2. **It is the best option because it is safe:** Dr. Sebi's cure is all-natural, and all the ingredients contained therein are devoid of any synthetic material. Herbs have been in existence since the time the very first man was made, and the reason they are still preferred over conventional medicine because they have zero side effects. Since Dr. Sebi's cure is entirely made up of herbs, you do not have to worry about your present and future health. These herbs work like magic, not only in curing you of herpes but also in improving your health every day. Those who have used Dr. Sebi's herpes cure in the past have backed up the claim that these herbs indeed improved their health as they felt more energetic after starting the course. This makes Dr. Sebi's herpes cure the only alternative you should consider.

3. **It is the best because it is cost-effective, too:** With antiviral drugs, you need a prescription. Dr. Sebi's herpes cure is different, as you do not need a prescription when you make a purchase. This alternative medicine is much less than the money that goes into consultation. Health is essential, but the money spent on antiviral drugs is excessive, which does not guarantee their effectiveness. On the other hand, Dr. Sebi's herpes cure is available in nature. You do not need to pay a consultation fee, and zero marketing cost is involved. You only pay for what you get. Since it is effective and gets the job done, you are not throwing away your hard-earned cash.

4. **It is the best because scientists certify it:** Dr. Sebi's claim to cure herpes with herbs has been verified by various medical and scientific research. Some of the studies established more facts about the herbs' antiviral properties used in the herpes cure. Natural antiviral properties can rid the body of the herpes virus without any side effects. In addition to the antiviral properties found in these herbs, they have also been found to be immune-modulatory. That means they directly boost the body's disease-fighting mechanism. A more muscular immune system means that the herpes simplex virus's replication can be put under control for every herpes patient to live a herpes free life. All the researches about Dr. Sebi's herpes cure approve it as the best solution for herpes.

5. **It is the best because it gives you herpes free life:** The efficacy of Dr. Sebi's herpes cure is the sole reason it is considered the best herpes treatment worldwide. No other treatment has been verified to cure herpes, only this one. You need to trust Dr. Sebi's methods to live a herpes free life.

The highlighted points are why Dr. Sebi's herpes cure is the best one around. If you think it is time to put an end to the pain herpes are putting you through, you should give this cure a try.

In the wake of taking a gander at the fixings, it is by all accounts all the more encouraging solution for herpes, isn't that so? Indeed, it can murder the herpes simplex infection. It has everything that is expected to help herpes patients carry on with a herpes free life. You may be on antiviral medications at present and can remain on the equivalent in the future too. Only for a couple of days, give this supernatural item a possibility, and you will never need to glance back at some other herpes treatment.

Herpes fix is a typical point encompassed with such a significant number of inquiries and no reliable answer. If you have herpes, your brain might be loaded with questions identified with herpes treatment. Herpes is a disease that is spreading worldwide; many individuals are influenced by herpes, yet with regards to herpes fix, nobody thinks about it. The ongoing revelation of herpes treatment is Dr. Sebi herpes fix.

This isn't just a name; however, the most anticipated comprehensive solution for herpes that can cause your fantasy about getting the chance to free of herpes work out as expected. Dr. Sebi is the author of the Dr. Sebi inquiry about foundation, which professes to fix illnesses like malignancy, A.I.D.S., lupus, diabetes, fibroids tumor joint inflammation, sickle cell sickliness, and now herpes as well.

Every one of these illnesses, including herpes, are the large difficulties for the human to deal with, and now it is an ideal opportunity to get an answer for every one of them. The sicknesses like herpes need more mindfulness and information because you deal with the successive episodes of herpes and control the transmission up partly with these. You ought to know about the infection; you can discover your responses for the herpes treatment at exactly that point.

The following steps were what Dr. Sebi used to cure herpes:

- Put an end to consuming acid foods. Ensure your body is not fed with acidic foods.

- Clean your body of acids and toxins and start eating alkaline diets and herbs that increase your cells' level of oxygen.

- Feeding your body with the needed nutrients can repair, rebuild, and completely strengthen your body at the cellular level.

- Practice fasting. Take herbs and water only during fasting. You can add green juice if the fasting becomes too difficult for you.

- Endeavor to eat foods from Dr. Sebi's nutritional guide after your body has been cured of herpes. Detoxification is at the heart of ridding the body of the herpes virus-there is no other way that will bring the necessary results."

-

Ways to cure herpes

Herpes and Alkaline diets

For the healing of herpes, an alkaline diet is needed. Dr. Sebi emphasized the significance of this and how important it is to eliminate 'blood and starch,' as he calls it, referencing animal flesh-like all sorts of animals, seafood, and starchy foods. However, it is essential to move beyond this when it applies to herpes recovery since even some of the things on Dr. Sebi's food list or dietary guide can be avoided. And why? Only that some of the ingredients are soothing better than others. Dr. Sebi stated that his collection comprises of 'least harmful' foods; nevertheless, you want food, which is as alkaline as possible and refreshing as possible. For this cause, fasting was believed to be such an essential factor in Dr. Sebi's recovery – it helped the body break from the ingestion of mucus-forming foods and acids; cleaning will begin, and the oxygen amount to the cells may improve.

An alkaline diet is essential for the whole process of herpes cure. On numerous occasions, Dr. Sebi stressed the vitality of avoiding what he calls "blood and flesh," that is, animal flesh, meats, fish, and starchy foods. When it comes to healing herpes, you need to go over and beyond by avoiding some of the foods on Dr. Sebi's list.

That is simply because some foods have more healing factors than others. Dr. Sebi has always referred to his food list as "least detrimental" as the diet is alkaline based, and it cleanses the body. That is the sole reason why fasting boosts this healing method's effectiveness as it allows the body to break acid consumption and begin the cleansing process.

During this time, alkaline herbs should be consumed in a high quantity as it helps cleanse and nourish the body and strengthen the immune system.

During this time, eat alkaline herbs to aid with detox and rejuvenate and recharge the body and improve the immunity.

What exactly you have to do?

1. Stop foods that are fried.

2. Delete all acid-forming items from the diet.

3. Take just the water and herbs for fasting (if you can't incorporate green juices).

4. Instantly, after a time of easy eating, only vegetables and fruit from the dietary guide also involve new green juices. Your leafy vegetables primarily contain green fluids. During cleaning and detox, the less stable the diet, the smoother and more successful the healing process.

5. Once you have eliminated herpes from the body, even then, keep consuming only items from the dietary guide.

6. Nuts, grains, and seeds must be avoided while recovering from herpes. Whereas mangoes, citruses, leafy greens, and berries are recommended.

When questioned, Dr. Sebi replied very correctly that the healing time depends on the degree of body toxicity, fluid, weight, and health condition. Everyone has a different stage of fitness, and therefore the duration of recovery differs, so the healing time varies between people.

You can detoxify herpes from a body, but the results also depend on how dedicated you are to the procedure. Herpes is not the most straightforward virus to get clear because it sets up residency in the central nervous system's spinal cord and often remains there inactive for an extended period. Your body needs to 'wake it up' basically and usher it back. The herpes virus must be inaccessible to the body. An alkaline body is essential to keep the body alkaline by washing and treating the body through alkaline plants and alkaline food and fasting to become rid of herpes. This is Dr. Sebi's method.

What Does the Dr. Sebi Diet Consist of?

Alkaline diets are those which do not contain foods that contain acids.

Acidic foods contain high acid content, and they are most times detrimental to human health. When there is an increased amount of acid in the body, infectious diseases find it easy to thrive, grow, and develop. Dr. Sebi does not encourage these kinds of foods in his diet, as they might hinder the effectiveness of his recommended herbal products and foods.

The Dr Sebi diet is a vegetarian, plant-based eating regimen and a basic eating routine (Source: National Institute of Health). While following the eating regimen, numerous additional take herbs to sustain the cell, help rinse them and recuperate them from many years of frightful eating.

Dr Sebi believes soluble nourishments to be "electric nourishments" for your cell, which are live and crude nourishments that are for the "recuperating of the country."

When all is said in done, **Dr Sebi separates nourishment into six classes:**

- Live

- Crude

- Dead

- Half breed

- Hereditarily changed

- Drugs

He used to say that you should concentrate on numbers 1 and 2 (live and crude) while avoiding 3 – 6. This incorporates maintaining a strategic distance from seedless organic products, climate-safe harvests, for example, corn, and anything with included nutrients or minerals, which can be hard for individuals thinking about that there are such a large number of crossbreed and hereditarily altered (G.M.O.) leafy foods offered in supermarkets.

As per Dr Sebi, foods prescribed for individuals who need to live sound incorporate ready organic products, non-bland vegetables, crude nuts and margarine, and grains. Verdant greens, quinoa, rye, and Kamut can likewise assume a huge job in the Dr Sebi diet.

Acidic foods, including meat, poultry, fish, or items containing yeast, liquor, sugar, iodized salt, or anything seared, carry negative impacts on the human body.

Supplanting acidic foods with electric choices will assist with mending you from the negative impacts that corrosive produces.

Following to a great extent, crude weight control plans can appear to be distasteful to acidic people. Yet, you gradually begin to become accustomed to a simple eating routine as you purge your cells of poisons, prompting the fix of the disorder.

Limiting corrosive in nourishments assists with diminishing bodily fluid in the body, which makes a soluble situation that makes it extremely hard for sickness to frame. Remembering herbs for your purging methodology is stunningly better.

Advantages of an Alkaline Diet

Weight Loss

This part is clear as crystal. Weight reduction will undoubtedly happen when following the eating routine because the Dr Sebi diet comprises regular vegetables, natural products, grains, nuts, and vegetables.

Immune System Boosting

A feeble resistant framework is the aftereffect of ailments and disorders. In some cases, they have fortified their insusceptible framework and have been recuperated from specific infirmities by following the Dr Sebi diet reliably. We, as a whole, realize that medication doesn't fix infections.

Decreased Risk of Disease

Acidic nourishments disintegrate the mucous layer of the cells and inward dividers of the body, which prompts an undermined framework that makes infection conceivable and a fix unimaginable. Subsequently, eating basic nourishments can lessen the danger of sickness and help your body get what it needs to take care of the great cells.

Vitality

Diets overwhelming in meat, dairy, and white sugar can delay your body and vitality levels. Concentrating on plant-based living is a superior approach and can improve the vitality that you show all the time.

Expanded Focus

Following Dr Sebi's lessons will assist with clearing cerebrum mist, keep you engaged and less disturbed by unpleasant circumstances that emerge.

Whether you are not wiped out, utilizing a plant-based philosophy will help you carry on with a long and solid life.

Alkaline Diet and Relationship with Herpes Virus and H.I.V.

Dr. Sebi said that an alkaline diet is essential for eradicating the herpes virus since it helps the body break any mucus-forming components and clean the body to the cell level.

This detoxifying process destroys the viral cells by making the body's environment inhabitable for them. Also, these viruses' oxygen content to grow, reproduce, and multiply will be removed. That makes the body filled with the necessary component required to fight disease.

Tips on Adopting the Diet

To adjust to the Dr. Sebi method for eating, you'll need to begin rolling out certain improvements to your general dietary patterns. You will probably find that to do this expects you to be in the correct outlook and enthusiastic state.

Be genuinely and intellectually arranged

Eating is a piece of regular daily existence, the sorts of nourishments and substances we expend everyday structure into solid propensities that can endure forever whenever left unchecked.

These propensities can be amazingly difficult to break or change; also, the impact of family and those nearest to us can, on occasion, be a block.

Along these lines, preceding racing into the Dr Sebi diet and way of life, you ought to invest some pondering changing your eating – don't guarantee yourself one or the other just to bomb because of absence of arrangement, family issues or whatever and break that guarantee.

Begin drinking more water

Water is basic to rinse our bodies, keep up sound cerebrum and body works just all in all host of different advantages.

Also, various of Dr. Sebi's items, for example, his Bromide Plus Powder, contain herbs, for example, Bladderwrack that have purgative impacts and elevate pee to expel poisons; along these lines, you should drink more water to renew this and keep yourself hydrated.

He recommends drinking up to one gallon of spring water every day. Springwater is prescribed because it is normally basic, not faucet water, high in chloride and different contaminants.

Add all the more entire foods to your current eating routine

Begin to remember all the more entire nourishments into your current eating routine for an everyday schedule.

This can be anything from your preferred natural product to a crisp filet of fish. The principle thought here is to devour all the more entire nourishments instead of bundled food sources brimming with added substances. Keeping away from these added substances will help you later on in your excursion; the same number of these things are addictive.

Refined sugar is incredibly addictive and makes us have food desires.

Begin perusing fixing names

It won't be simple for the vast majority to surrender certain nourishments or soda pops. However, an extraordinary method to begin is to peruse nourishment fixing marks.

That is a decent propensity and a flat out need to remain aware of what you're eating and drinking. Before all else, while you are not eating dependent on the healthful guide, this mindfulness will give you the impetus to change your propensities as you progress.

Later, when you do begin to receive the eating routine, on the off chance that you do wander, you can, in any case, keep aware of what you ate.

Eating the correct way

Eating can be a significant urgent propensity; however, that doesn't mean it must be an awful one. The vast majority like a nibble from time to time; however, instead of going after a pack of chips, why not make your path blend of pecans, raisins, and other dried natural products if you need some fast and simple couch snacks.

Dr. Sebi's Products for Herpes

Dr. Sebi developed five effective herbal products that have helped a lot of people to treat herpes.

These supplements are:

A.H.P. zinc powder

The term A.H.P. stands for ayurvedically herb purified. The purification of zinc is done with decoctions of natural herbs such as Aloe Vera to produce A.H.P. zinc powder.

- A.H.P. zinc power is of a better benefit than the usual zinc tablets you consume. A.H.P. zinc powder is prepared from naturally occurring zinc, making it very easy for your body to absorb.

- A.H.P. zinc powder also has the main qualities of some of the herbs used in preparing it. Modern medicine also acknowledges the importance of zinc for herpes treatment, but it is better to use A.H.P. zinc powder instead of zinc tablets.

- A.H.P. zinc powder is safer and more effective in treating herpes.

- A.H.P. is also known as ayurvedic herbs purified.

- A.H.P. zinc powder is gotten from zinc that occur naturally, and this natural currency zinc is very easy for your body to absorb. Also, the naturally occurring zinc is healthier than the usual off counter zinc.

- A.H.P. effectively treats the herpes virus, repairing damaged skin, and treating sores and blisters.

The potency A.H.P. zinc powder includes:

- It helps reduce and fight inflammation.

- It is instrumental in healing cold sores and wounds.

- It helps heal skin infections.

- It promotes the healthy growth of your cells.

- It helps boost your immune system and help your body to fight off diseases.

- It contains powerful antiviral properties.

Triphala

Triphala contains three outstanding herbal combinations.

The three herbs that makeup Triphala are:

- Harad

- Amla

- Baheda

- These three herbs have not only been acknowledged for their potency by Dr. Sebi, but other medical experts have conducted research on these three great herbs and praised their efficacy.

- This herbal combination is a good combination that can be taken by both healthy persons and people that have the herpes virus.

- This herbal combination can clean the unwanted materials and toxins in your body and help purify your blood and many organs.

- Dr. Sebi didn't only administer this herbal combination to his patients but also took it daily for optimal health and longevity.

- Triphala is a powerful herb containing three crucial herbal combinations: amla, bibhitaki, and haritaki.

- Dr. Sebi recommended these three herbal combinations that make up the Triphala to treat the herpes virus.

- Medical experts also acknowledged it because of its potency and efficacy.

- These herbal combinations can also help purify and cleanse your body and remove toxins from your bloodstream.

The potency of the Triphala herb includes the following benefits:

- It helps heal cold sores, blisters, and wounds.

- It is useful in reducing inflammation.

- It contains powerful antioxidants that quicken the healing of cold sores and blisters caused by the herpes virus.

- It has potent antiviral properties.

- It helps eradicate skin infections.

- It prevents bloating.

Pure Extract Giloy Tablets

- Pure extract giloy tablets are produced manually from the extracts of the best quality Giloy. The Giloy used to make these tablets is gotten from the best quality Giloy.

- Giloy is the perfect herb to improve your immunity and fight sexually transmitted diseases (S.T.D.s)

- Dr. Sebi himself was a big fan of Giloy, and now, modern medical experts have accepted that Giloy can help your body fight off many diseases and improve health.

- The giloy herb contains powerful antiviral properties that help boost your immune system and fight viral infections such as the herpes simplex virus and sexually transmitted diseases.

- Giloy contains powerful properties that can be useful to treat the herpes simplex virus and boost your health.

These properties are:

- Giloy extract is a potent antiviral agent.

- Giloy extract helps cold sores and blisters to heal faster.

- It helps reduce inflammation.

- It helps boost your immune system and help your body fight off infection.

A.H.P. Silver Powder

- Ayurvedically herbs purified (A.H.P.) is a process that involves purifying various minerals in herbal decoctions, making them useful for medication,

- A.H.P. ensures that the minerals maintain their excellent abilities and absorb the herbs' nutrition and qualities, which they are purified into.

- A.H.P. powder is exceptionally helpful to your health, especially your nervous system. Dr. Sebi administered A.H.P. silver powder to several of his patients with herpes, and the results were always good.

- What makes A.H.P. silver powder effective for herpes is that it works on your neurons. The very place where the herpes virus in your body use as it's home and hiding place.

- A.H.P. silver powder works by sending silver nanoparticles into your neurons to eliminate and flush out the herpes virus in your neurons.

- Once you have completed your fast, you would need to take fruits and vegetables to improve the healing process.

- Once your herpes is gone, you would need to continue with the Dr. Sebi recipes for a while to keep you healthy and make the healing process a permanent one.

- Herpes is curable, as we know with all we have learned from Dr. Sebi, and it can be done on a budget as well. You do not need to spend a fortune to get this done, and all you have to do is follow the simple process highlighted here.

- For Dr. Sebi's herbs for herpes to work effectively for you, you have to start with the cleansing herbs.

- A.H.P. silver powder effectively treats the herpes simplex virus because it targets your nervous system, which is the infection's hidden point in your body.

- This powder performs the function of eradicating the herpes simplex virus from your body by sending silver nanoparticles into your nervous system to flush out the herpes virus.

- It contains potent and effective antiviral properties to treat cold sores, flu, and the herpes virus.

The Potency of A.H.P. Silver Powder include:

- It contains a potent antibacterial property that enables it to eradicate the herpes simplex virus from your body.

- It has antibacterial properties.

- It helps reduce inflammation that prevents the herpes simplex virus from healing.

- It quickens the healing of cold sores and blisters.

- It helps eradicate skin infections.

Punarnavadi Mandoor

- Punarnavadi mandoor is not a herb purified mineral, but a healthy herbomineral created from the combination of herbs and minerals.

- Punarnavadi mandoor is an extraordinary combination of healthy minerals such as calcium, iron and great herbs such as shunti, punarnava, alma, etc.

- This herbomineral combination works perfectly on the liver and helps to eliminate toxins in the liver.

- Dr. Sebi administered this herbomineral combination to many of his patients, and the reason for this is that the liver's function was disrupted during infection. Punarnavadi Mandoor is the perfect option to bring the liver function back to normal.

- Punarnavadi Mandoor is a healthy and nutritious herbomineral prepared naturally from herbs' combination, and not an ayurvedicallly herbs purified mineral.

- It is a combination of naturally occurring minerals such as iron, zinc, and calcium. It also contains powerful herbs like Alma, purnarnava, and shunt.

- The herbal combination is advantageous in removing toxins from your body and cleansing your blood.

- Dr. Sebi recommends taking this herbal combination because he discovered that the liver function is disrupted during viral infection, thereby making healing impossible or slow. So, the purnarnavadi Man door helps restore the liver to its normal position and quickens the healing process.

The potency of Punarnavadi Mandoor includes:

- It helps reduce inflammation that blocks the healing process of the herpes simplex virus.

- It contains powerful antiviral properties that help to heal the herpes virus.

- It heals blisters, cold sores, and wounds.

- It helps eradicate skin infections and other infections in the body.

- It contains powerful antibacterial properties.

Dr. Sebi Alkaline foods to help fight Herpes

Almost all of the alkaline-forming foods could be considered superfoods. It isn't just because of their ability to help the body keep a healthy pH balance, but also because of nutrient density. Alkaline forming foods are plant-based and have many healing properties.

You might know that it is very healthy to drink warm lime water or fresh green juices. They can improve the body's ability to detox, boost the immune system, and give you a massive dose of nutrients. That is because all of these can help raise the body's pH level, which turns your system from being acid to alkaline.

If you were a good student during chemistry class, you might remember the concept of alkali and acid. Acids will have a pH level of less than seven, where alkalis will have a pH level of greater than seven. Water is the most neutral, with a pH of seven. This means that acids will be corrosive in nature and sour in taste. Alkalis will be used to neutralize acids.

It will become more disease resistant that inhibits the growth of organisms such as cancer, fungi, yeast, viruses, and harmful bacteria. The oxygen levels get raised in our blood, organs, and tissues. That enables them to function more efficiently and effectively. It can reduce the acidity and keep the alkaline state that encourages toxin excretion, energy production, and healthy cell turnover.

The easiest way is by what we eat. When we eat alkaline-forming foods and minimize how much acid-forming foods we eat, our bodies can keep up the alkaline state. An alkaline-forming food will be plant-based and are rich in antioxidants, minerals, and vitamins. These are easier to digest, improving the gut's immune function, and helping lower mucus production and inflammation.

While our bodies are digesting our foods, the stomach secretes gastric acid. It helps to break down the food. Our guts will have a pH of between 2.0 and 3.5. That is very acidic, but we need it to be able to digest our foods right. But, there are times when because of bad food habits or bad lifestyle choices, the acid level gets haywire, and this can cause gastric ailments, acid reflux, and other problems. Suppose you were to look at the regular diet of any American. In that case, it will contain vast amounts of acidic foods like pastries, doughnuts, colas, kebabs, bacon, sausages, cheese sandwiches, rolls, pizza, samosa, burgers, and many more that could cause the acidic balance in our stomachs.

When these foods get broken down, it leaves behind a residue that is called acid ash. That is the chief cause of stomach problems. Foods that are acidic once our body digests them are processed foods, refined sugars, whole grains, eggs, dairy products, and meats. You need to know that a food's alkaline or acid tendency doesn't have anything to do with the food itself. Limes are acidic but do have an alkalizing effect on our bodies. Alkaline foods are needed to bring our bodies in balance. Like many doctors and experts have said for years, we need to have a balanced meal with everything instead of restricting ourselves to eating one food category. Alkaline foods can help counter the risks of acid reflux and acidity, bringing us some relief.

Here is a list of the best alkalizing foods that are versatile and delicious. These can be used alongside any other alkalizing vegetable or fruit to help cleanse the body from toxins that are slowly killing us.

Kale

There is an excellent reason that kale has been called the new beef. It is high in vitamin K, calcium, and plant iron. These can help protect you against some cancers.

Kale is mild in flavor and can kick up any recipe. You can add it to any smoothie that calls for greens. Add it to soups, salads, and stir-fries for an excellent alkaline boost.

Cherries

they are a great source of antioxidants like anthocyanins that can prevent cancer. Studies have shown that cherries can help with inflammation associated with arthritis and joint pain. They could even help prevent cardiovascular disease.

Cherries can be put into any smoothie. They are great in a post-workout shake because they contain protein and alkalizing nutrients.

Any post-workout smoothie needs to include alkaline foods because lactic acid gets released when you exercise. Lactic acid helps increase energy. Lactic acid makes the body more acidic; this is why it is essential to eliminate the acidity by eating more alkaline foods after you exercise.

Pears

These beautiful fruits are low in sugar but high in fiber. It makes them an excellent fruit for anyone who has blood sugar problems. They are high in vitamin C, which in turn helps protect cells from carcinogens.

Zucchini

It is an excellent source of phytonutrients like lutein. Lutein is in the same antioxidant family as beta carotene, which means it has better benefits for protecting your eyesight.

Zucchini is now a trendy vegan, gluten-free, low carb pasta alternative. Zucchini noodles are easy to make by using a spiralizer that you can find pretty much anywhere.

It is easy to throw together a quick zucchini pasta but pairing it with basil, other spices, and vegetables.

Apples

they have always been considered to be the healthiest food around. That is because they are full of antioxidants like vitamin C, detoxifying fiber, and flavonoids that can protect you against cancer. These nutrients are great for helping with cholesterol and high blood pressure.

Try adding them to dishes you normally wouldn't consider putting them into to get more benefits from your apples.

Watermelon

they give our bodies essential electrolytes for heart health like potassium. Because watermelons are made up of mostly water, they can help keep you hydrated better than other vegetables and fruits.

Watermelon is an excellent snack by itself, but it is fun to be creative. Make a smoothie out of watermelon, ginger, agave syrup, and a dash of cayenne.

Other Leafy Greens (Dandelion, Amaranth, Turnip, and Sea Vegetables)

Almost all leafy greens will have an alkalizing effect on our bodies. It isn't any wonder that our ancestors and doctors always tell us to eat out greens. They have essential minerals that are needed for our bodies to carry out their functions. You can add sea vegetables, turnip greens, amaranth greens, and dandelion greens to any smoothie or meal.

Key Limes

Most people think that since limes are highly acidic, they would have a cutting effect on our bodies, but they are an excellent alkaline food. Limes are also loaded with vitamin C and can help detoxify our bodies while giving relief from heartburn and acidity.

Sea Salt and Seaweed

it has about 12 times more minerals than greens that are grown in the ground. They are very alkaline food and can give your body many benefits. You can add in some kelp or nori to your stir fry or soup. Using sea salt as your main seasoning can bring more alkalinity to your body.

Walnuts

Many people love to munch on walnuts when they feel hunger kicking in. Other than being a great source of healthy fats, they create an alkalizing effect in our bodies.

Onion

including red onions, which are an essential ingredient in Indian cooking, and they bring lots of flavor to your dishes. If you cook them in a healthy oil like avocado oil, it will increase their alkalinity. Eating them raw is an excellent choice since onions have many nutritional benefits other than being alkaline-forming. They have antibacterial and anti-inflammatory effects and are full of vitamin C. You can use them in many different ways to spice up your tea, soup, or stir fry.

Tomatoes

These will be at their most alkalizing when raw. Tomatoes do contain many nutrients, whether natural or cooked. Eat a sliced tomato as a snack with a sprinkle of sea salt, or add it to your favorite omelet or salad.

Avocado

It is a powerhouse of deliciousness and nutrients. Avocados contain lots of healthy fats, plus they are heart-healthy, anti-inflammatory, and very alkalizing.

Basil

it is the tastiest alkalizing ingredient. It is high in calcium, vitamin K, and vitamin A. It is high in flavonoids with antioxidant effects.

Mushrooms

they contain antioxidants, minerals, vitamins, and protein. They can have many benefits for our health. Antioxidants are chemicals that can help keep our bodies get rid of free radicals.

Free radicals are byproducts of bodily processes and metabolism. They get trapped in our bodies, and if too many are trapped, oxidative stress could happen. It could harm the body's cells and can lead to many health problems.

Mushrooms contain choline, vitamin C, and selenium. The antioxidants in mushrooms could help prevent breast, prostate, lung, among other kinds of cancers. They can also help with heart health, diabetes, and pregnancy. They are high in B vitamins like niacin, pantothenic acid, thiamine, folate, and riboflavin.

Foods to avoid

Acidic foods:

Acidic foods are not good for the healing of herpes. Foods with high acidic levels are not good for herpes infection. These foods can open up the cold sore before it heals, and this prolongs the healing period. So, avoid foods like juice, soda, etc. You may consider taking water as a substitute until the sickness heals.

Arginine

Chocolate and some other foods high in L-arginine should be avoided. L-arginine is known to prolong the healing of the herpes virus.

Sugar

Instead of taking added sugar, one can easily go for oranges, mango, bananas, etc. Added sugar is usually converted to acid in the body.

Processed Foods

By maintaining a low level of oxidative stress, you can naturally quicken the healing process. Processed foods may promote oxidative stress due to synthetic preservatives.

Alcohol

Studies have shown that alcohol can suppress white blood cells. It means that alcohol can make the body susceptible to infections.

FAQs

1. Why Women Stand a Greater Risk of Getting Infected with Genital Herpes?

One of the reasons is the way women are made. The genital area has a large number of mucosal cells, i.e., cells that contain body fluids.

Another reason is the menstrual cycle. This cycle change affects the immune system. A lower immune system makes it easier for the herpes virus to create an infection.

2. How Do Women Contact Genital or Vaginal Herpes?

Women contact herpes just the same way men do. The fluids released by the HSV-1 and HSV-2 all contain the virus that causes herpes.

3. What Are the Parts of Healings?

Whether it is arthritis, HIV, or dementia, there are two necessary steps to healing known as the cleansing/detoxifying of the body and revitalizing it.

4. What Is the First Thing to Consider for Healing Herpes?

Anyone suffering from herpes means that he is suffering from a weak immune system. So, the first thing to consider is how to build back the immune system to work correctly again.

5. What Are the Food to Avoid While Treating Herpes?

Avoid eating inflammatory food like amino acids as they help feed the herpes virus, leading to a flare-up. Foods like sugar, processed foods, and animal products (meat and dairy protein).

6. What Are the Basic System or Structure That I Need to Cleanse to Heal Herpes?

Based on what late Dr. Sebi states, the only way to get rid of disease and live a sick-free life is by cleansing the following structure through intracellular cleansing. It doesn't matter what condition you want to get rid of, and the steps remain the same.

That is, cleansing of:

- Gallbladder

- Lymph gland

- Liver

- Kidney

- Colon

- Skin

Dr. Sebi's diet herpes cure is anchored on some facts. Let us look at some of those facts that made Dr. Sebi's diet for herpes cure so effective:

1. **It is a plant-based alkaline diet. It** is designed to eradicate acidity from the body and is effective in purifying and detoxifying the body.

2. **It strengthens the immune system** and prime the body to fight off diseases such as the herpes virus.

3. **It helps eliminate mucus, heal an already compromised mucus membrane, and empower** your body to heal itself of diseases such as herpes.

Chapter 5: Dr. Sebi's 3-Step Method

Detoxification and Cleansing

As I said before, Dr. Sebi thought that every disease's source is the excess of mucus that slowly builds up in different parts of our bodies because of the acidic environment the 'standard' diets create.

As Dr. Sebi stated, human bodies can face six stages of over-acidity if the body its not nourished with alkaline foods and herbs:

1) **Sensitivity** ➔ You know you are in this stage if you start suffering from low energy, acne, or bad odor.

2) **Irritation** ➔ The next one is where you start facing bowel diseases such as IBS, constipation, diarrhea, or skin problems

3) **Mucous Formation** ➔ Here's where your body can't tolerate to live in an extra-acidic environment anymore and start producing mucus to try to protect itself

4) **Inflammation** ➔ As soon as the mucus starts to build up, your body reacts by starting the inflammation process. That might cause you to start suffering from Arthritis or Fibromyalgia

5) **Indurations** ➔ This stage's most dangerous complication is Atherosclerosis, also known as "the hardening of arteries". When mucus starts depositing into them, it takes the name of 'plaques'. Over time, these plaques can narrow or block the arteries and causing unforeseen problems, as strokes.

6) **Degeneration** ➔ In the last stage, mucus starts to build up into the brain, bones, and around nerves. If that happens, dangerous diseases may arise, such as cancer, Multiple Sclerosis, or Osteoporosis.

As strategies to remove pollutants from the body, reduce weight, or improve wellbeing, several "detoxification" or "cleansing" regimens have been introduced.

The words cleanse & detox are also used synonymously, and although both eliminate contaminants from the body, two separate items are a detox and a cleanse. It is clean at the core of the term "cleanse," and you must think of washing as a way to clean the body. To specifically remove toxins, cleanse frequently utilizes vitamins or tablets, and cleanses typically concentrate mostly on the digestive system. Detox services, on the other side, aim to help the normal toxin-eliminating cycles in the body. Because the liver & the kidneys are the key detoxing centers in the body, successful detox programs concentrate on helping the kidneys and liver by supplying them with the vitamins and nutrients they have to operate optimally.

What are poisons anyway, then? Heavy metals are top of the mind, like arsenic. However, chronic chemical contaminants, chemicals, & pesticides are still included in the report. Toxins are simply toxic compounds that will reside in the bloodstream, disturbing cells, triggering irritation, & interacting with the body's usual functions.

Indications of toxins or a heavy toxin load (and hence the need for detoxification or cleansing) provide the following:

- fatigue

- headaches

- joint pain

- depression

- anxiety

- constipation

The Cleansing Journey

Making the stomach safe is linked with cleansing. The digestive system is the system the body receives its nutrients from. It becomes inefficient in performing out its tasks as it gets unstable. In the stomach, the pile-up of the dump will turn poisonous, contributing to pain and disease. Bloating is among the symptoms of a dysfunctional stomach. When the body cannot get rid of waste as it can, that's due to gas accumulation. The food continues to decompose then. Food, as meant by default, must be natural and organic.

There are both positive and destructive microbes in the digestive system. It contributes to problems if the equilibrium of such bacteria is disrupted. Purging, in which a laxative is used to eliminate human waste, parasites, and other such unnecessary material, is the essential cleansing method. The concern with this technique is that it would be non-selective & clears up the harmful benefits. It may also be harmful since, during the phase, you may lose extra water, which would make you drained. One of its reasons is that the body system gets a strip of toxic chemicals to consume lots of water.

A vice president & dietician of the Sports Education Society, Marie Spano, claims that workouts and adequate sleep play a vital role in making your function on the detox regimen.

Through curing the gut by taking note of what goes through it, a healthy way to detox is to practice regularly. It's considered fast food, and it doesn't have the nutrition your body requires. Instead, clogging things up appears to screw with the digestive tract. Soy, gluten, dairy, sugar, & caffeine-containing foods can be removed and substituted with unprocessed agricultural substitutes & additives.

The method of cleansing is not only complete with the clearance of waste from the digestive system. By supplying nutritious food that makes the gut function at its peak, it should be cured. That requires balanced food with adequate nutrition, which tends to maintain the stomach's safe levels in the stomach, such as good bacteria—organic beverages, such as unflavored probiotic yogurt, often aid.

Minneapolis Running's Sara Welle speaks about the advantages she gained as a competitor from the cleansing plan. You must go through a well before-cleanse process to start the detox method, where you'll have to strip out alcohol & different highly processed foods. Her program's early days were unpleasant. However, she noticed that her stress levels became much greater as the system matured and began to operate properly.

The Detox Route

Another approach to clear the body of destructive chemicals is to detox. Normally, through the liver, skin, and kidneys, the body requires the removal of pollutants. Detox can strengthen the contributions of these organs. So, what toxins are attacked by the process? For example, there are contaminants in the atmosphere you breathe in that make their way through your bloodstream, where they settle and create pain. Chemicals such as toxins, preservatives, & additives are still used in many products. During this time, meat must be avoided.

One of the actors whose detox was performed with is Gwyneth Paltrow. Over a 21-day duration, it is circulated. It's named The Safe Method by the psychiatrist who developed it. To clear the contaminants' body, he recommends a diet of shakes, nutritious foods, and vitamins—any of his patient's record post-program weight loss.

Your skin is often loaded with a mixture of chemicals hidden on the lotions of creams and other products you use. Often, the organs associated with detoxifying get overloaded. The detox can be supported by lemon, garlic, spinach, pineapple, and ginger. As several may have detrimental consequences, you can address them with a nutritionist. For starters, garlic thins the blood, which may threaten someone whose blood doesn't easily coagulate. Health supplements, too, aid enhance the health of the liver and kidneys.

What Are The Dr. Sebi Approved Detoxification/Cleansing Approaches?

Many detoxification programs are offered in an integrative health care model. The following are the approved methods to eliminate toxins in your body:

- Water Fast

- Liquid Fast

- Smoothie Fast

- Fruit Fast

- Raw Food Fast

Why You Should Detox

Detoxing or detoxification is a process of ridding the body of toxins and other harmful substances that have accumulated through time. Most toxins come from the food we eat, but they can also enter the body through the air we breathe and the medicines we take. Regardless of how these toxins came about, they can be harmful to the body and pose serious threats that need to be addressed if you want to stay healthy and at your peak.

Weight Loss

Weight loss is one of the biggest reasons why people go through detoxification or why they even think about the idea. Detox for weight loss is fairly straightforward and easy to understand, as this involves eating natural and unprocessed foods. That means less, or even no, junk foods and unhealthy food options make you put on those extra pounds. Going on a detox diet means taking in fewer calories and, therefore, potentially losing weight if coupled with a good exercise program. While weight loss is perhaps the most publicized benefit of detox, most detox programs involve short-term solutions that lead to short-term results. Detox can help you lose weight, but most especially if you make it a regular part of your lifestyle.

Boosts Energy

Many detox programs result in increased energy levels for participating individuals. While it is hard to quantify energy or just how much of it a person has, the results pretty much speak for themselves, as people who undergo detox programs generally feel more energetic. They report feeling less sluggish and having an overall feeling of just wanting to be out and about and doing things rather than just lying around all the time. That can be attributed to the fact that detoxification releases the toxins that lower the body's energy levels.

By steering clear of the things that provide toxins such as sugars and trans fats, the body is free from such substances' sluggish effects. Moreover, replacing such negative foods with natural energy boosters such as fruits and vegetables can increase a person's energy levels in the best way possible. Added to this is that detoxification means keeping the body hydrated at all times, resulting in more energy and better efficiency when performing daily tasks.

Stronger Immune System

The health benefits of detox or detoxification also include a stronger immune system. Toxins are naturally harmful to the body, or at the very least, they prevent the body's systems from functioning the way they should be. By going through cleansing programs that rid the body of these toxins, the different systems can function more efficiently and effectively. The immune system specifically is given a boost, allowing a person to be less prone to sicknesses and diseases once detoxification has been completed.

The removal of toxins allows the body to absorb nutrients better, including Vitamin C, vital for the immune system. A stronger immune system and the removal of harmful toxins and contaminants help the body fight off diseases more easily. Furthermore, detox programs make use of herbs that help the lymphatic system function better.

What Are the Benefits of Dr. Sebi's Detoxifying Process?

- Provides energy for the body.

- Revitalize the body.

- Remove toxic waste from the body.

- Multiply cells in the body.

- Provide the body with irons, which is very important for the cure of the herpes virus.

- Cleanses and promotes blood.

How Many Days Does It Take to Cure Herpes Virus?

In one of his lectures, Dr. Sebi stated that the sufferer's weight and health condition would determine the number of days it will take to be cured. The curing time for an individual varies as everyone has a different health condition.

He also stated that the liver, gut, body fluids, and pancreas' health condition would determine how long it will take a sufferer to achieve a complete cure from this disease.

Furthermore, practice fasting; plan it and go for it. The more you fast, the quicker you receive your cure. You can consume dates if you are very weak during fast.

Dr. Sebi's Official method for getting rid of herpes, such as any other disease, is composed of 3 main steps. Please note that any of these parts CAN'T be passed over to succeed in your healing journey.

<u>**The three steps I'm talking about are:**</u>

1. **Cleansing ➔** The body must be cleaned on an intra-cellular level through detoxification to purify each cell and remove mucus excess.

2. **Revitalizing ➔** After cleansing, you need to nourish your body to regenerate your cells and strengthen the immune system.

3. **Avoiding Outbreaks** → Follow Dr. Sebi's nutrition guide and adopt healthy lifestyle habits every day to keep your mind and body in good shape.

Cleansing

How to Prepare Cleansing Herbs?

Preparing your cleansing herbs would depend a lot on the form you purchased them. It's easier to prepare cleansing herbs in powder forms, as you can easily make herbal teas with them in the specified or recommended dosage. However, for other forms form herbs, especially roots or leaves, it is better to use a ratio of 1 teaspoon to 1 cup (8 oz) of spring water for each herb.

However, for easier batch preparation and storage, I recommend preparing herbs in batches of mixtures. That would mean mixing them up according to function and benefit. Again, this will depend on the state of your health and what minerals are most important for you. You can combine similar herbs with similar functions into a batch. Like our healer, Dr. Sebi would say: *"If you want calcium, you know where to go to (sea moss), if you want Iron, you go to Burdock, and if you want a mix of both Iron and Fluorine, you go to Lily of the Valley".*

In all, try not to mix more than 2 or 3 herbs. Remember, these herbs are electric, and it's best to preserve their organic carbon, hydrogen, and oxygen nature as much as we can. Again, if you mix more than that, you may not get their accurate concentrations per ml of water, so try to limit it to 3, possibly 2.

For a clearer understanding, you can use the following mix:

- Mix **Colon and gallbladder** cleansing herbs together

- Mix **liver and kidney** cleansing herbs

- Mix **respiratory and mucus cleansing** herbs

- Mix **lymphatic and heavy-metal** cleansing herbs.

Since these herbs perform a whole-body cleanse (not just colon), including the skin, eyes, colon, liver, lymphatic system, and gallbladder, you can decide to choose how to combine them. Also, note that when you make larger batches of these herbs for storage, try not to make batches that last more than 7 to 14 days.

For pre-purchase cleansing packages

Please follow the recommended dosage or instructions that are provided for that cleansing package

For fresh Green leafy herbs

- Place in spring water and boil on low heat for 5 to 7 min

- For dried leafy herbs, boil longer – 10 to 15 min

For Dried ground (or powder) herbs

For dried ground or powder leaves or roots, mix in recommended ratios for the herb. Powder herbs are the easiest to mix in dosage proportions, so you can simply follow the package instructions

For Chunks of Dried Root herbs

If you've purchased chunks of roots or stems, you can prepare them in the following way:

- Cut or break up chunks

- Place in spring water and boil for 15 minutes

- Let cool and serve

- Alternatively, prepare in larger batches and place in jars to store in the refrigerator.

For bulk purchase herbs

If you have purchased herbs in bulk and you're making your teas, find out what the recommended dosage is for each herb. As a general rule, you should prepare each herbal tea ratio of 1 teaspoon to 8 ounces of spring water.

For capsules

I recommend that you do research and find out what the recommended dosage is for each herbal capsule

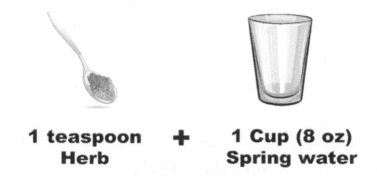

1 teaspoon + 1 Cup (8 oz)
Herb   Spring water

How To Take The Prepared Cleansing Herbs

If you are on medication, I recommend taking the herbs one hour before taking your meds; Dr. Sebi recommended this. Your colon cleansing herbs should not be consumed for longer than 30 days because your body may become dependent on them, and you want to start to reduce the dose during your last 3 to 5 days, depending on how long you've been taking them.

Routine:

- **Twice a day** - morning and night

- **Daily Consistency** - Try to stay consistent both in terms of timing and duration. That is, try not to skew the duration. Make it consistent, and take the cleansing herb throughout the cleanse. For example, for a 14-day cleanse, the cleansing herbs can be taken twice daily, and you should take them around the same time you do take them on both mornings and evenings.

- **Gradual Wean Off** – Just like medications, it is not the best to go cold-turkey when it comes to herbal detox. Towards the end of the cleanse duration, wean off your herbs by gradually reducing the dosage and duration. The duration of the wean will depend on the length of the fast you choose. For example, for a one month fast, I usually start weaning a week towards closure. For a 14 day fast, I begin weaning on day 11 or 12. You can begin the wean by reducing it from twice a day to once a day. Or simply take half the dosages each for mornings and night.

You must do this because you need to signal your body to begin to prepare to start functioning independently without dependence on herbs' cleansing. And no other way to do this than to take it slow and gradual, without bringing too much "shock" to your body.

Cleansing Herbs

Mullein

Mullein is a flavorful beverage flowering plant that has been used for centuries to treat various ailments. Research shows that this herb is an effective anti-microbial, anti-inflammatory, anti-cancer, anti-hepatotoxic, antioxidant, and anti-viral herb with potency to prevent a lot of health disorders. It helps to cleanse and detoxify the lungs and lymph system and destroy cancer.

The benefits of consuming Mullein include:

- It helps treat and prevent various types of cancer by destroying cancerous cells and preventing them from mutating.

- It helps to eliminate mucus from the small intestine

- It helps to activate healthy lymph circulation in the chest and neck

- It helps neutralize the negatives effects of free radicals by protecting the cells from damages caused by free radicals.

- It helps treat and prevent various bacterial and virus infections like herpes viruses, HIV etc.

- It helps to treat and prevent respiratory tract infections.

- It helps to treat and prevent tuberculosis.

- It helps to treat earache.

- It helps to treat various health disorders like bronchitis, stroke, heart diseases etc.

- It helps to prevent some chronic brain diseases like Alzheimer's, Parkinson's etc.

- It helps to treat atherosclerosis and others in the biological systems.

- It helps to treat and relieve pain that is caused by inflammation and tumor.

- It also helps treat various ailments like asthma, bronchitis, migraine, congestion etc.

When writing this book, there are no negative side effects attributed to mullein consumption by mouth; But, since there is no information to show that this herb is harmful or not to pregnant and breastfeeding mothers, I advise them to avoid its consumption.

When writing this book, there are no medications that interact with mullein as it can be combined with other herbs and drugs without any issues.

Quantity Needed and Procedure

For the dosage and how to prepare Mullein tea/infusion, kindly take the following steps:

1) Get some handful of fresh Mullein from a nursery farm or garden and dry it, or you can order for a prepackage Mullein tea bags online.

2) Once the new leave is dried, pour some cups of water in a saucepan and boil it.

3) Once the water is boiling, measure 8.12ounce or 240ml of the boiling water, add a handful of Mullein dried leaves to the boiling water, and steep it for 20–25 minutes.

4) Please keep it to get cold and strain it using a strainer or filter to remove the tea leaves.

5) For the dosage, if you are using the flower, take 3–4g of mullein flowers daily, and if it is the fresh leaves, take 15 to 30 mL of fresh leaves 2–3 times daily.

Eucalyptus

The eucalyptus tree is a fast-growing evergreen tree that is a native of Australia. This plant's leaves and bark are used for various medicinal purposes like joint and muscle pain, cold, cough, congestion, etc. However, the Chinese, Greek, and Indian Ayurvedic people have incorporated this amazing herb to treat various types of conditions for thousands of years before now.

This plant/tree has more than 400 different species. The most used is the Eucalyptus globulus or the Australian fever tree, also known as Blue Gum.

Eucalyptus leaves cineole that is also known as eucalyptol, in which the leaf's gland contains essential oil (eucalyptus oil) and also; flavonoids and tannins, which are plant-based antioxidants that aids in reducing inflammation, control blood sugar, fight against the activities of bacteria and fungi and the oil can help in relieving pain and inflammation as well as blocking chemicals that usually cause asthma.

The benefits of using or consuming eucalyptus tea/infusion include:

- It helps in cleansing the skin through steaming/sauna.

- Eucalyptus helps in relieving common cold symptoms like cough lozenges and inhalants and also sore throat and sinusitis

- It helps in relieving symptoms of bronchitis. Inhaling the vapor of eucalyptus tea helps serves as a decongestant by loosening phlegm and easing congestion.

- It aids in relieving asthma: research showed that eucalyptus has the potency to break up mucous in people who have asthma.

- It aids in dental plaque and improves gingivitis: research carried out on eucalyptus shows that eucalyptus leaf has the potency to reduce dental plaque and improve gingivitis.

- It helps in improving bad breath: research showed that eucalyptus has the potency to improve bad breath.

- It also helps to relives some health like; skin disease, bladder diseases, gallbladder and liver problems, bleeding gums, diabetes, burns, ulcer, stuffy nose, wounds, etc.

The precaution to be note-full of before using eucalyptus tea or infusion include:

- It is 100% safe for pregnant and breastfeeding mothers to consume eucalyptus tea/infusion, but the oil is unsafe.

- The tea is safe for children, but the oil might lead to seizures

- Because of eucalyptus leaves' potency leaves to lower blood sugar levels, it is advisable to consult with your doctor before using the tea with any diabetes medication

Quantity Needed and Procedure

For the dosage and how to prepare eucalyptus tea/infusion, kindly take the following steps:

1) Boil water to (90-95)0 or 194-205 Fahrenheit. Alternatively, you can boil the water and drop it down for a minute or two to reduce the temperature.

2) Pour a teaspoon of dried eucalyptus leaf into a teacup/mug.

3) Pour 6 ounces of water (from the first step) inside the teacup/mug and allow the leaves to be steep for 10-15minutes. (you can enjoy breathing the vapors of the steeping tea)

4) Get a filter to strain the loose leaves of the eucalyptus.

5) You are a god. You can now enjoy the cup of eucalyptus tea/infusion at a go.

6) For the dosage, take 3-4 cups per day.

Kale

Kale is a cruciferous vegetable family member, including broccoli, Brussels sprouts, arugula, and collard greens.

Some of the benefits of consuming kale are listed below. For example:

- It is loaded with powerful antioxidants, such as quercetin and kaempferol, that have powerful heart-protective, blood pressure-lowering, anti-inflammatory, anti-viral, anti-depressant, and anti-cancer effects

- It is one of the world's best sources of vitamin C. A cup of raw kale contains even more vitamin C than a whole orange.

- Kale contains bile acid sequestrants, which can lower cholesterol levels. It might lead to a reduced risk of heart disease over time

- It is one of the world's best sources of vitamin K, which is critical for blood clotting, and does this by "activating" certain proteins and giving them the ability to bind calcium

- It is also a good source of important minerals that most people don't get enough of, such as calcium, potassium, and magnesium

- Being a high nutrient-dense food, with a low-calorie and high-water content, kale provides significant bulk that helps make you feel full and avoid overeating

Precautions and Side Effects

- Consuming too much kale, which is high in potassium, can be harmful to people whose kidneys are not fully functional.

Red clover

Red clover, scientifically known as *'Trifolium pratense'*, is a wild plant belonging to the legume family. It has been used medicinally to treat several conditions, including cancer, whooping cough, respiratory problems, and skin inflammations, such as psoriasis and eczema.

Below are some of the main benefits of this herb:

- It lowers the loss of bone mineral density in postmenopausal women

- It may help reduce the risk of prostate cancer

- It may help relieve the discomforts of menopause, especially hot flashes

- It has also been used as a cough remedy for children.

How to prepare Red Clover tea/infusion:

- Add 4 grams of dried flower tops to 1 cup (250 mL) of boiling water

- Steep for 10 minutes

- Enjoy!

Note: it's best to limit your daily intake to 1–3 cups.

If you relate to any of these symptoms during the cleansing stage, be happy. That's because your body is pushing out all the toxins and mucus you have been keeping inside for so long. These symptoms are only temporary and usually resolve after the first one to two weeks.

Burdock Root

Burdock root is the root of a delicious plant called Burdock, which all its body or parts are useful as either food or medicine. This plant can be found all over the world. I called this plant the wonder plant because everything about it is important as we consume its root as food, and we also use it for medicinal purposes, and both its leaf and seed are used for medicinal purposes.

For over five centuries, people worldwide have been using burdock root orally to treat and prevent various health disorders.

Because of Burdock root's chemical composition, such as; quercetin and luteolin, research has it that it can serve as a great effective antioxidants that can treat and prevent cancer by preventing cancerous cells from growing and mutating and also combat aging. Compound like 'Phytosterols' helps boost scalp and hair follicles to grow healthy hair even from baldhead. The vitamins-C helps in boosting the immune system and combat bacterial. It also helps to cleanse or detoxify the liver and lymphatic system, etc.

The potassium helps reduce blood sugar levels and filter the blood by removing impurities through the bloodstream and eradicating toxins through the skin and urine.

The benefits of using or consuming burdock root tea/infusion include:

- cleanse/detox the liver and lymphatic system.

- Treat and prevent diabetes by reducing blood sugar levels in the body.

- Eliminate toxins from the body by inducing sweetness and urine.

- Purify the blood by removing heavy metals from the bloodstream.

- Treat various skin disorders and combat aging.

- Treat and prevent cancer by inhibiting the growth and mutation of cancerous cells.

- Boost the immune system and enhance circulation.

Till at the time of writing this book, there are no side effects that have been recorded by researchers or people that have used these herbs.

However, research has it that applying this root to your skin might cause rashes.

Quantity Needed and Procedure

For the dosage and how to prepare Burdock root tea/infusion, kindly take the following steps:

1) Scrub the uprooted root of burdock heartily under running water to remove all the dirt that accompanied it from the soil.

2) You should chop the Burdock root into smaller pieces (less than 1 inch). Please note that if you order it online, it will come dried and already chopped.

3) Pour 2-3 cup of water into your saucepan and add ¼ cup of the chopped burdock root and boil it.

4) Once the water is boiling, lower your gas, re-boil it for 30-40 minutes, and put off your gas.

5) Once it is cold, strain it and consume it.

6) For the dosage, drink one glass cup daily

Chaparral

Chaparral, also called 'Larrea Tridentate', is an herb from the creosote bush, a desert shrub native to southern areas of the United States and northern regions of Mexico. This flowering plant has bright yellow flowers and thick green leaves layered with a resinous coating. However, despite its pretty appearance, chaparral is a controversial herb that's even banned in many countries. However, this herb is claimed to help treat many ailments, including cancer, arthritis, and skin conditions.

The consumption of Chaparral has several benefits, such as:

- It contains a powerful antioxidant that helps the shrinkage of tumors

- It may prevent the spreading of HPV and HIV

- It prevents heart diseases by reducing levels of free radicals

- It helps to boost the immune system

- It relieves joint and muscle pain thanks to its anti-inflammatory quality

The Side Effects and note-full precautions before Consuming Chaparral are:

- Nursing mothers should avoid this herb because it has been reported to have abortifacient effects

- Although chaparral is a potent antioxidant, it has been found to have serious negative health effects, including hepatotoxicity, which is a chemically-induced liver injury

Quantity Needed and Procedure

For the dosage and how to prepare Chaparral tea/infusion, kindly take the following steps:

1) Boil water to (90–95)0 or 194–205 Fahrenheit. Alternatively, you can boil the water and drop it down for a minute or two to reduce the temperature.

2) Pour a teaspoon of dried chaparral leaf into a teacup/mug.

3) Pour 6 ounces of water (from the first step) inside the teacup/mug and allow the leaves to be steep for 10–15minutes. (You can enjoy breathing the vapors of the steeping tea).

4) Get a filter to strain the loose leaves.

You can now enjoy the cup of the chaparral tea/infusion at a go.

Dandelion

Dandelion is a flowering plant known as 'yellow gowan' or 'lion's tooth'. This plant is native to Eurasia and today. It is common in over 60 countries worldwide in the mild climates of the northern hemisphere. For centuries, these flowering plants have been used for the treatment of swelling (inflammation) of the pancreas, relieve pains that are caused by inflammation, treat and prevent cancer, tonsils (tonsillitis), skin disorder, bladder or urethra disorder, digestive and liver problems and enhance the general health of the liver and digestive system.

Researchers proved that it is a very effective cleansing/detoxification herbs because of the chemical compositions and nutrients.

The benefits of using or consuming Dandelion include:

- It helps to detoxify or cleanse the liver and the kidney.

- It helps to treat and prevent diabetes by regulating blood sugar levels.

- It helps to fight against and relieve pains that are caused by inflammation.

- It helps to deactivate and inhibit the negative effects of free radicals in the body, which is because of its antioxidant properties.

- It reduces the level of cholesterol.

- It helps to naturally shed excess weight gain by improving the metabolism of carbohydrates.

- It helps in boosting the digestive system.

- It helps to boost the immune system.

- It helps to keep the skin healthy and treat and prevent skin diseases.

The special precautions before using/consuming dandelions are:

- Pregnant and breastfeeding mothers should stay off dandelion as there is no research to know if it is harmful to them or not.

- If you are suffering from Eczema, stays off dandelion as more than 85% of people with eczema suffer an allergic reaction to dandelion.

Quantity Needed and Procedure

For the dosage and how to prepare Dandelion tea/infusion, kindly take the following steps:

1) Get some fresh leaves of dandelion and washed them under running water to remove all the dirt.

2) After washing it, pour ½ - 1 cup of the washed dandelion into your saucepan.

3) You should boil 4-5 cups of water and pour the boiled water inside the saucepan where you pour the dandelion and cover it for 12-15 hours or throughout the night (overnight).

4) The next day, strain out the dandelion leaves, and you will be left with the dandelion tea/infusion.

5) For the dosage, take ½ tablespoon of Dandelion per ¾ cup of water three times daily. And if you ordered your dandelion online, you can take 4-10 grams of dry leaf of dandelion three times daily.

Elderberry

Elderberry is a dark purple berry from the elder tree, also known as European Black Elderberry or Sambucus Bacchae. This plant is a flowering plant from the family of Adoxaceae and native to Europe. Both the leaves and fruit (berries) of elderberry have been used for centuries to treat pain and swelling arising from inflammation. It also helps to stimulate urine production and induce sweat to detoxify the body system.

Because of how rich elderberry is with various compounds and nutrients like vitamin-C, dietary fiber, phenolic acids, which is a great and powerful antioxidant that helps to prevent and decrease the damage that is caused by oxidative stress in the body, it also contains some compound like flavonols such as kaempferol, quercetin, isorhamnetin and anthocyanins which gives the fruit the black-purple color and makes it a strong antioxidant and anti-inflammation agent.

Elderberry also contains some nutrients, like:

- Calories

- Carbs

- Minute amounts of protein and fat

- And anthocyanins, making the plant a strong and effective antioxidant with anti-inflammatory properties.

The benefits of using/consuming elderberry include:

- It helps cleanse and detoxify the lungs and respiratory system by eliminating mucus from the upper respiratory system and the lungs.

- It helps to treat constipation.

- It helps to treat flu and cold in less than 24hours.

- It combats harmful bacteria in the body by preventing bacterial growth through its antibacterial properties.

- It boosts and supports the immune defense system by increasing white blood cell production.

- It protects and keeps the skin healthy.

- It helps to relieve chronic fatigue syndrome and depression.

Till at the time of writing this book, there is no record of any side effects from researchers and people who have used elderberry, but because of the compound that are presents in elderberry, it will be wise to use it for not more than 12 weeks and take a break for at least a week before using it again.

The special precautions before using elderberry include:

- Ensure children below 12 years do not use/consume elderberries, and children above 12 and less than 18 should not use it for more than 10days.

- Since there is no reliable information to know if elderberries are safe or not for pregnant and breastfeeding mothers, I strongly advise that they stay off elderberries.

- People who have a history of suffering from an autoimmune disease like; multiple sclerosis, lupus, rheumatoid arthritis, etc., should stay off elderberry as it has the potency to boost the immune system become more active, which could worsen their situation.

- Since elderberries have the potency to increase or boost the immune defense system, any medications designed to decrease the immune system's function will certainly interact with Elderberry.

Quantity Needed and Procedure

For the dosage and how to prepare Elderberry tea/infusion, kindly take the steps below:

1) Boil 8-12oz of water in your saucepan.

2) Once the water is boiling, measure one tablespoon of dried elderberries and add it to the boiling water.

3) Reduce your gas and allow it to boil for at least 15 minutes.

4) After the 15 minutes timing, allow it to get cold and strain it using a strainer.

5) For the dosage, consume 3-4 cups daily.

Elder Flower

Both the berries and the elder plant's flowers have been used for medicine for thousands of years. While both have similar affinities for boosting the immune system and fighting off infection, elderflowers have some unique uses.

Some of the benefits of consuming elderflower are listed below. For example:

- It is widely used for colds and flu, sinus infections, and other respiratory disturbances due to its antiseptic and anti-inflammatory properties.

- It also has diuretic and laxative properties and helps relieve occasional constipation

- Elderflowers have relaxing properties.

- It is rich in bioflavonoids, mostly flavones and flavonols, that are most commonly known for their antioxidant

- It has antibacterial and antiviral properties

- It can be used for its antiseptic properties as a mouthwash and gargle

<u>Some special precautions before using elderflower include:</u>

- **Pregnancy and breast-feeding**: There isn't enough reliable information to know if elderflower is safe to use when pregnant or breast-feeding

- **Diabetes**: If you have diabetes and use elderflower, be sure to monitor your blood sugar levels carefully.

- **Surgery:** Stop using elderflower at least two weeks before a scheduled surgery.

One thing that seems certain is that you should not brew up any other part of the elder tree. The leaves, sticks, and roots can cause a build-up of cyanide levels in the body.

<u>Quantity Needed and Procedure</u>

For the dosage and how to prepare Elderberry tea/infusion, kindly take the steps below:

1) Put Loose Elderflower Tea into a tea infuser

2) Brew fresh water using either filtered or bottled water.

3) Place the Tea-filled accessory into a cup or mug.

4) Fill the cup with hot water

5) Let it infuse for 5-10 minutes

Cilantro

Cilantro is a popular herb around the globe that comes from the 'Coriandrum sativum' plant. It resembles flat-leaf parsley at first glance, but it transports you to the Mediterranean, Mexico, Asia, and India at first sniff. In some parts of the world, people call it 'coriander'.

Some of the benefits of consuming cilantro are listed below. For example:

- It has been shown to bind arsenic, aluminum, and mercury together (which are toxic metals), loosening them from tissue and facilitating their elimination from the body.

- A recent study has shown that due to its natural sedative properties, this herb can help calm the nerves and improve sleep quality, almost at the same level as the popular medication Valium

- A study published in the *International Journal of Food Microbiology* found that cilantro is particularly protective against 'Salmonella', a bacteria that often causes what we know as food poisoning

- Its leaves and steams help lower blood sugar levels and improve overall health

- Its antibacterial compounds could help keep the urinary tract healthy and free from unhealthy bacteria in an alkaline environment.

- Thanks to its antioxidant properties, cilantro may help protect your brain from serious disease such as Alzheimer's and Parkinson's

Quantity Needed and Procedure

For the dosage and how to prepare Cilantro tea/infusion, kindly take the steps below:

Ingredients

- 1 cup water

- 3 sprigs of cilantro

Instructions

1.   Boil the water in a kettle or on the stovetop. Pour it into a teapot.

2.   Steep the cilantro leaves in hot water for 5-7 minutes.

3.   Remove the leaves, and drink!

How to break a detox fast?

- Slowly reintroduce solids

If you are doing water or a liquid fast, you will need to reintroduce solid foods slowly. You can begin by introducing solids like high water-content fruits. These include watermelon, apples, and berries. After that, you can proceed to introduce softer fruit solids like bananas and avocados. Later, you can incorporate more harder solids like veggies. All foods must be listed on the nutrition guide. However, if doing a fruit or raw veggie fast, you can break the fast right away on solid foods.

- Drink 1-gallon spring water daily

Drink spring water daily together with the revitalizing herbs and sea moss.

How long should you detox/cleanse?

How long you should detox depends on your state of health, that is, your body's toxification level (the less healthy you are, the more toxic your body is) and tolerance level. Typically, it is recommended to fast for 7-14 days, but Dr. Sebi recommends a minimum of at least a 12 day fast. Dr. Sebi himself fasted for 90 days to cure himself of diabetes, asthma, and impotence. It is great to cleanse at least once a year for seven days if you consume an alkaline diet. If you are not consuming an alkaline diet, then you should cleanse/detox every three months

I fasted for 14 days, and I would recommend fasting for between 14 days and one month if you have high blood pressure. Again, your body's tolerance level will ultimately determine the length so, watch your body and study its reaction as you begin the fast. We are all different, and you may find that you cannot handle a basic liquid fast (water or juice). In that case, you can get started with fruit or raw vegetables fast. But make sure all foods and fruits are listed in the Dr. Sebi Nutrition Guide. Whether liquid, juice, or raw food fast, the results are virtually all the same – the only major difference is when it takes to begin to see results. While raw food fasts take longer, liquid fasts are much faster. So do not worry; the most important thing is to stay committed and focused on whatever fasting method you choose.

Common Symptoms Expected During Detox Cleanse

- Cold and Flu symptoms

- Changes in Bowel movements

- Fatigue and Low Energy

- Difficulty sleeping

- Itching

- Headaches

- Muscle aches and pains

- Acne. Rashes and breakouts

- Mucus expel (catarrh, etc.)

- Lower blood pressure

If you relate to any of these symptoms during the cleansing stage, be happy. That's because your body is pushing out all the toxins and mucus you have been keeping inside for so long. These symptoms are only temporary and usually resolve after the first one to two weeks.

Revitalizing Herbs

These are herbs, oils, foods, and things of that nature that will target the herpes virus specifically. I also recommend that you take the revitalizing herbs after your detox.

So, when you are detoxing, you'd want to take your cleansing herbs and things like that to clean your body out. Then you'd want to reintroduce the revitalizing herbs - this is when you're eating your alkaline foods and things like that. You would want to go ahead and take the revitalizing herbs. However, if your body can handle a prolonged fast, you can take the revitalizing herbs after you have done your cleanse and then take that while you are still fasting, and it should give you faster results. But you want to make sure that you are taking your sea moss during that time to rebuild up some of the things you have flushed out during your cleanse that are beneficial to your body. Revitalizing herbs are herbs and oils that target the herpes virus specifically. It is important you take these revitalizing herbs after cleansing and detoxifying your body so that the herbs can completely clean your body.

Pao Pereira

Pao Pereira is a tree that belongs to the Apocynaceae family and native to South America. This tree's bark is very rich with various compounds that effectively destroy, eliminate, and inhibit cancerous cells. Because of how effective this tree's bark is, Dr. Sebi recommends this herb to revitalize the body system after cleansing.

The benefits of consuming Pao Pereira include:

- treating malaria and other infections caused by parasites.

- It effectively suppress the Herpes Simplex Virus

- It helps treat and prevent cancer by destroying cancer and preventing cancerous cells from mutation.

- Soothing and relieving liver pain.

- It helps to treat and prevent stomach disorders like constipation and irritation.

- It helps to boost sexual arousal

Till at the time of writing this book, there is no any side effect that is attributed to the consumption of Pao Pereira; but since there is no vital information to show that this herb is 100% safe for pregnant and breastfeeding mothers, I advise that they avoid this herb's consumption.

For the dosage and how to prepare Pao Pereira tea, kindly take the steps below:

- Harvest some Pao Pereira by cutting some of its bark without cutting down the tree, chopped it, and dried it.

- Once it is dried, boil 1liter of water and pour two tablespoons of the dried Pao Pereira into the boiling water.

- Lower the heat of the fire to a medium-low and place the lid on the pot.

- Boil the mixture under medium temperature for 20 minutes.

- Allow it to get cold and train it using a strainer or filter.

For the dosage, consume 1 cup of the tea times daily.

Pau d'Arco

Some of the benefits of consuming Pau d'Arco tea are listed below. For example:

- It has the power to naturally reduce pain in patients suffering from serious conditions, such as cancer

- It helps in fighting Candida

- It inhibits pancreatic lipase, an enzyme that helps the body better digest and absorb fat

- It has a strong antioxidant property that protects against oxidative damage triggered by inflammation

- It works as a detoxifier since it has a laxative effect

- It has been used for thousands of years as an antiviral herb, effectively fighting Herpes, Leukemia, and AIDS.

Side Effects

- If eaten in high quantity, it may cause some issue like: nausea, vomiting, and anemia

Quantity Needed and Procedure

For the dosage and how to prepare Pau d'Arco tea/infusion, kindly take the steps below:

1) Put 2 tsp of barks into 3 cups of boiling water

2) Let it sit for 15 minutes

3) Let it cool for at least 1 hour

4) Strain the water

5) Enjoy your tea!

Holy Basil

This green leafy plant, also known as 'queen of the herbs' or 'tulsi', is native to Southeast Asia. Still, it has a history within Indian medicine as a treatment for many conditions, from eye diseases to ringworms.

Some of the benefits of consuming holy basil tea are listed below. For example:

- It helps prevent certain respiratory illnesses ranging from cold and cough to bronchitis and asthma

- It helps in maintaining normal levels of cortisol hormone, which correlates to stress and anxiety

- It is widely used to treat gastrointestinal disorders and menstrual cramps

- It helps with adrenal fatigue, which can trigger herpes outbreaks

- It helps combat against harmful bacteria and germs in the mouth

- It has anti-inflammatory properties that may help in relieving chronic pain

- It facilitates the metabolism of carbs and fats, ensuring that the blood's sugar is utilized for energy.

Side Effects

- If consumed in high quantities, it may temporarily decrease fertility in both men and women

- It is recommended for women to avoid consuming tulsi tea while breastfeeding

- When consumed in high quantities, some people may experience nausea or diarrhea

Quantity Needed and Procedure

For the dosage and how to prepare Holy basil tea/infusion, kindly take the steps below:

- Boil 1 cup of filtered water

- Pour it over 1 tsp of fresh leaves, ½ tsp of dried leaves, or 1/3 tsp of powder

- Cover and let it steep for at least 20 minutes

- Strain the leaves, and enjoy!

Blue Vervain

Blue Vervain is a perennial flowering plant that belongs to the family of Verbenaceae. It is rich with various nutrients like iron fluorine, which purifies the blood, phosphorus, phosphate, zinc, potassium, magnesium, etc. Because of this potency, Dr. Sebi recommends this herb for revitalizing your body after cleansing.

The benefits of using or consuming Blue Vervain include:

- It helps to treat and prevent anxiety and sleeplessness and enhance mood.

- It helps to treat and calm the central nervous system.

- It helps to soothe the nerves and relaxes the mind, thereby treating migraine headaches.

- It helps boost and protect the heart's health, treat and prevent myocardial ischemia, chest pain, and heart failure.

- It helps to fight against both internal and external inflammation.

- It helps to treat menstrual cramps or pain and stomach pain.

- It improves digestive health and protects the livers and kidneys by cleansing/detoxifying both the kidney and liver.

The note-full precautions before consuming blue vervain tea include:

- Because there is no information to show if these herbs are good for breastfeeding mothers or pregnant women, I advise that they avoid these herbs' consumption.

- Till at the time of writing this book, there are no medications that interact with blue Vervain.

Quantity Needed and Procedure

For the dosage and how to prepare Blue Vervain tea, kindly take the following steps:

1) Get some fresh leaves and flowers of blue Vervain and dry them.

2) Once it is dried, pound or chopped it, or you can order it online, and it will come dried and chopped.

3) Boil a cup of water (8ounce) in a saucepan.

4) Once the water is boiled, pour it into a cup, measure 1 teaspoon of the Blue Vervain, and add it to the water.

5) Allow it to steep for 10-15 minutes and strain it.

6) You are done! For the dosage, take 2-4 cups daily.

Sarsaparilla

Sarsaparilla root is the root of a tropical wood climbing vine that belongs to the genus Smilax family. Dr. Sebi recommends it as a revitalizing herb for many diseases, including cancer, because it is rich in iron, calcium, and phosphate.

The benefits of consuming Sarsaparilla roots are:

- It helps to destroy and prevent cancerous cells from mutating.

- It binds the endotoxins responsible for the lesions in psoriasis patients and eliminates them from the body system.

- It helps to fast-track healing and recovery.

- It treats and prevents health issues that are caused by inflammations like: joint pain, swelling of any parts of the body, arthritis, rheumatoid, etc.

- It soothes and heals sexually transmitted diseases such as syphilis, herpes, gonorrhea etc.

- It helps to treat and prevent leprosy

- It helps to protect and reverse damages done to the liver to function perfectly.

- It makes the body absorb nutrients and other herbs easily

Quantity Needed and Procedure

For the dosage and how to prepare sarsaparilla root tea, kindly take the following steps:

1) Get the root of fresh sarsaparilla.

2) After getting it, pill it and remove the outer skin.

3) You should now dry the outer skin in a well-ventilated place (indoors), but it will come dry if you are getting it online. So you won't have to disturb yourself with these steps.

4) Ensure you turn the root daily for 6–7 days to dry it until it is completely dried.

5) Ensure that you store your dry sarsaparilla in a paper bag or cardboard box once it is dry.

6) For the dosage of Sarsaparilla root, boil water and add 1–4 grams of sarsaparilla root in 8–12oz of the boiling water and allow it to simmer for 15–20 minutes.

You are good. You can now enjoy your sarsaparilla root tea/infusion three times daily.

Guaco

Guaco is a climbing plant with different names like Huaco, Guace, or Vejuco. This climbing plant belongs to Asteraceae and cordifolia species' family and is very rich in numerous minerals and compounds. Its leaves are very medicinal and nutritional, that the people of Aztecs use them for cleansing the blood system and clearing heavy metals from the bloodstream.

There are a lot of benefits that one can benefit from using or consuming Guaco. Some of them are:

- It lessens the effect or symptoms of snake poison.

- It is used to thin the blood through the coumarin activities it contains (anticoagulant and blood-thinning.)

- It helps to combat inflammation through its anti-inflammatory properties.

- It treats stomach irritation through the effect of its cleansing activities.

- It helps to treat respiratory disorders like coughs, rheumatism, bronchitis, etc.

- It enhances quick recovery from the wound.

- It helps to cleanse or detoxify the blood and skin by clearing heavy metal from the blood.

- It boosts and builds the immune defense system.

- It can treat some infections diseases such as; candida yeast infection, herpes, etc.

Quantity Needed and Procedure

For the dosage and how to prepare Guaco tea/infusion, kindly take the following steps:

1) Get some handful of fresh Guaco and wash it under running water or 2 ounces of it dried leaves if you have the dried ones.

2) Pour about 6cups of water in your saucepan together with the Guaco leaves boil it until it is reduced to 2 cups.

3) You can add some brown sugar (optional) if you count the brown sugar; allow it to boil for another 20 minutes.

4) Strain the syrup with a strainer.

5) It would help if you bottled it and stored it in a refrigerator.

For Guaco dosage, take one soupspoon 3–4 times daily.

<u>**When Should I Start Consuming the Revitalizing Herbs?**</u>

The best time to consume the revitalizing herbs is the next day after you finish your cleanse. For instance, if you fast for 14days, on the 15day, you should start consuming your revitalizing herbs.

<u>**What Are the Things That I Shouldn't Forget?**</u>

- Drink at least a gallon of spring water daily.

- Once you are done with your detox /cleanse, eat foods only on Dr. Sebi's nutritional guide.

- Never forget to use sea moss during the revitalization process

- Ensure you do an intra-cellular cleanse once per year for at least seven days if you follow only the alkaline diet from Dr. Sebi's nutritional guide. Still, if you are not, you should always do an intra-cellular cleansing after every three months to cleanse your body from mucus and toxins.

Please note that consuming acidic food can only put your body at the risk of outbreaks.

Herbal treatments with Dr. Sebi essential oils

Some Dr. Sebi herbs are highly effective when used in the treatment of herpes. They work well by speeding up the healing process, numbing discomfort, and relieving itching.

These herbal products are used as essential oils and should be handled with utmost care. If essential oils are not diluted, they can burn through the skin. So, it's advisable to dilute them with carrier oils such as coconut oil. Also, the mixture should be tested before use.

Steps to test essential oil solution

- First, apply the mixture to the firearm.

- Wait for about 24 hours.

If there is no adverse effect on the skin, you can then go-ahead to use it. But if you notice any negative effect, please discard it and never use it.

Essential Oils made from Dr. Sebi Approved Herbs

Olive leaf extract

Herpes is an illness brought about by an intelligent infection (Herpes Simplex Virus), which will, in general, play so savvy in the body that it is never get captured by any medication neither the safe framework. It turns out to be extremely hard to fix this ailment and isn't a simple errand to do. Be that as it may, there has been exploring distinctive approaches to fix Herpes, one of which incorporates Olive Leaf extricates.

Olive leaf separate originates from the leaves of the olive plants. The concentrate contains phenolics, for example, oleuropein, which keeps up glucose digestion and skin wellbeing. It is said to be perhaps the best fixing to fix herpes. It is said to have mending powers and has been utilized for treating different ailments as well.

Olive leaf removes are assembled from the Olive plant, which contains hostile to viral, mitigating, against tumor, hostile to microbial, cell reinforcement, and progressively different properties. Olive leaf separate is a cure that battles a wide range of infections. It has been demonstrated to be a superior strategy than other drugs that don't influence well-being. It has been demonstrated to be powerful to fix the Herpes.

The compound called Oleuropein tends to execute the available infections. Herpes begin developing in our framework when our insusceptible framework gets feeble by stress or when our body neglects to deliver protein. Oleuropein present in the Olive leaf is the primary segment that battles the infection and secures the invulnerable framework.

Even though herpes doesn't dispense with appropriately, it helps in forestalling the infection to episode further. When we devour the olive leaf, it assaults and harms the infection in our body and forestall further reason. Along these lines, the odds are less of the infection getting repeat; however, it will most likely experience the host's demise.

Instructions to Use Olive Leaf Extract for Herpes:

- Three to four tablets of before 6 hours of your supper. The dose must be just a single tablet at regular intervals.

- Take the prescription until you see a change

On the off chance that a change happens, that implies the medication is working. If you take a greater amount of the tablets, you will confront certain side effects like weakness, influenza, migraine, and so forth.

Take less measure of tablet on the off chance that you see manifestations and on the off chance that these side effects don't leave; at that point, quit taking the tablets.

See a specialist that will set up a legitimate calendar for taking the medication and will likewise tell the best way to take it and what the progressions that will happen will fix.

You can join olive leaf removes with Aloe Vera, which can upgrade the activity for quicker outcomes.

You can likewise utilize Oregano Oil with olive leaf extricate together for better-restored results.

How Much Of Olive Leaf Extract Should I Take?

The olive leaf contains oleuropein, which contains 20 mg that aids in better assimilation and expels the infection that causes herpes in our body. That is the best home-grown drug one can settle on. Some olive leaves are not transformed into cases. They are dried, and afterward, they are placed in a glass of warm water and devoured legitimately. That is useful in restoring herpes. 500 mg must be expended every day and that too four times each day. You are to take dried leaves per drink alongside the tablets on the off chance you need to expend three times each day.

Are There Any Side Effects of Using Olive Leaf Extract?

There is no such damage, yet more utilization may prompt minimal symptoms. The overdose may make the infection increasingly confounded and may prompt genuine disease. The prescription must be taken appropriately since it might mess the heart up when a greater amount is taken. The heart may diminish its pulsates, and circulatory strain may go down. It may likewise bring detoxification issues simply like: Diarrhea, Nausea, and so on. In this way, legitimate consideration must be taken.

If one experiences brevity of breath, a quick move should be made as many individuals can be touchy towards a specific type of oil like olive oil.

So, we can reason that the olive leaves are the best medication for restoring herpes. The dried leave or the cases both give an advantage to the body and assault the infection of herpes. An appropriate amount must be taken to guarantee great wellbeing.

Lavender oil

Lavender oil contains aggravates that are disinfectant, antibacterial, and hostile to contagious. That essentially implies Lavender executes and represses germs and infections.

If you have a virus bug experiencing your home or office, at that point utilize Lavender

Essential oil to help stop it. Diffuse it into the air to clean and filter the air and stop those airborne germs.

That is such a great amount of more advantageous than to splash however frightful unpronounceable synthetic disinfectant showers. Those by themselves could make you wiped out!

Lavender likewise inspires one's temperament, and this will enable the insusceptible framework to help its safeguards.

Approaches to Help Stop the Germs Using Lavender

You can add drops to a splash container of water and spritz down territories of transmission, for example, the telephone, door handles, and counter. Dry with a spotless material.

Diffuse it in an Aromatherapy Diffuser to chop down the airborne germs and to inspire the feelings.

Oregano Essential Oil

Oregano essential oil is antiviral, best at 90% concentrate. Anything less than 90% will not benefit you that you need to heal from the herpes virus. You'd want to apply it to your lower spine, which is where the HSV2 herpes virus is dormant. It can also be applied under the tongue as well as to the genital area. You would want to use it two to three times per day. I recommend you put ten drops into two ounces of extra-virgin olive oil, or you can also use coconut oil because you want to dilute this, or it will burn your skin. Oregano essential oil is a great antiviral that can suppress the herpes virus. It works best at ninety percent concentration. Apply essential oregano oil to your lower spine because your lower spine is the point where HSV-2 is dormant. You can also apply it to your genital area and under your tongue. Oregano essential oil is a great antiviral that can suppress the herpes virus. It works best at ninety percent concentration. Apply essential oregano oil to your lower spine because your lower spine is the point where HSV-2 is dormant. You can also apply it to your genital area and under your tongue.

Ginger Essential Oil

You can also use ginger essential oil. It is very similar to the effects of oregano oil; it can kill the herpes virus on contact. It must be diluted as well with a carrier oil.

How to Extract Essential Oils for Herpes?

There are numerous oils for herpes. The one thing that we have to consider is the extraction process.

The proper extraction of these oils from their natural sources is a delicate process that requires a lot of experience and the right materials.

There are numerous methods of extracting essential oils. Still, we are going to cover the two most important techniques, which are:

Steam distillation

The process of steam distillation makes use of steam and pressure for the extraction process. This process is a simple one, but without the right expertise, it can go wrong.

The raw materials are placed inside a cooking chamber made of stainless steel. When the material is steamed, it is broken down, removing the volatile materials behind.

When the steam is freed from the plant, it moves up the chamber in gaseous form through the connecting pipe, which goes into the condenser.

Once the condenser is cool, the gas goes back into liquid form, and this is the essential oil that can be collected from the surface of the water.

Cold Pressing

The cold press process extracts oils from the citrus' rind, and the seeds oil the carrier oil. This process requires heat but not as much heat as the steam distillation process with a maximum temperature of 120F for the process to go as planned.

The heated material is placed in a container where it is punctured by a device that rotates with thorns. Once puncturing is complete, the essential oils are released into a container below the puncturing region. These machines then make use of centrifugal force to separate the essential oil from the juice.

Both processes are essential. It has to be done properly with the right level of information from experts who know a lot about the process; if not a lot of harm, good can and will be done.

Avoiding Flare-ups

Once you can no longer see any of the symptoms you suffered from, you can consider the 'Revitalizing' process ended. At this point, you need to focus on living your life the healthy way, following the Dr. Sebi nutritional guide to avoid outbreaks and maintaining your body in its natural alkaline state, where disease can't manifest itself.

I'll give you some lifestyle tips to living a herpes-free life, but before that, let's see 4 of the most common factors that may trigger a flare-up:

- **Sexual intercourse** ➔ As for genital herpes, some people find that the friction of sexual intercourse irritates the skin and brings on symptoms. Using a water-based lubricant can help reduce irritation.

- **Sunlight and Colds** ➔ Exposure to sunlight or cold may trigger flare-ups of cold sores (HSV-1)

- **Weak Immune System** ➔ People whose immune system is weakened by HIV or chemotherapy, for example, tend to experience outbreaks more often

- **Hormone Imbalance** ➔ Quick hormonal changes, like those that occur in women during the menstrual cycle, may cause genital herpes outbreaks.

Most importantly, the number one factor that correlates to herpes outbreaks is stress.

Managing stress is the number one thing you need to focus on to avoid flare-ups, implied by the fact that you will follow the Dr. Sebi nutritional guide and eliminate over-acidity from your body.

Here are five lifestyle tips you can follow to manage stress better and keep herpes away:

Sleep enough

When you don't get good sleep, you drain your entire body and brain of vital functioning energy. In response, your body and brain are reduced to anxiety; it may be hard for you to focus and make logical thoughts. On the other hand, anyone experiencing an anxiety episode is advised to get a maximum of 8 hours of uninterrupted sleep. I know I say 8 hours, and it may be hard even to make them fall asleep. What you can do, try and prepare the environment in which they will sleep in, make it cozy, warm, and secure; you can even sleep by their side so that they know you are there. When you do all these, the person's brain starts adjusting from anxiety mode to relief mode, and thoughts like, 'I think I am safe in this room, I think she will make me safe' is what will be crossing their minds.

Exercise

While exercise has been clinically proven to reduce anxiety and improve mood, it can also treat many other health problems. Health issues can be a major anxiety trigger, and easing the symptoms of those ailments can further reduce anxiety symptoms.

Also, exercising can help people relax. When a person exercises, their body releases hormones that produce a calming effect. Exercise also increases body temperature, which can be very relaxing. Working up a sweat is tiring, but it's a great way to calm down.

When some people hear the word "exercise," they picture a gym full of lifting weights. However, many fitness activities can provide the exercise someone with anxiety needs. Even everyday activities like gardening or washing a car can elevate the mood.

Many people think they don't have time for exercise, but exercise doesn't have to take hours. Instead, people can find little ways to increase physical activity throughout the day. They might stretch at their desk at work or take a quick walk during their lunch break.

Studies suggest that 30 minutes of exercise a day, three days a week can dramatically reduce anxiety symptoms. However, those same studies show that even small amounts of activity can have a positive effect. If someone doesn't have time for lengthy workouts, they should still find ways to exercise their body needs.

While increase physical activity provides several health benefits, they aren't lasting. For exercise to improve anxiety, it must be done consistently. That makes it all the more important for people to find exercise routines they can stick with and physical activities that they enjoy.

For many people who suffer from anxiety, beginning an exercise routine is the hardest part. However, once they get started, they find these physical activity periods to be one of the most enjoyable parts of the day. Sticking with an exercise routine can be very easy if that routine is planned out well.

Anyone beginning an exercise routine should think about the physical activities they enjoy most. Do they enjoy playing with their children? Riding a bicycle? Gardening in their backyard? When it comes to reducing anxiety symptoms, any activity that gets the body moving counts as exercise.

No one should feel as though they have to decide on a workout plan and stick to it forever. Sampling a variety of different activities can help keep motivation levels high. Different kinds of exercises have different benefits, and switching between them gives people the chance to experience them all.

If the thought of joining a gym is enough to bring on a panic attack – you're probably not alone. You don't need to have a social phobia (or any other kind of anxiety disorder) to have an aversion to the gym! However, healthy exercise has some surprising implications for anxiety disorders and other psychological conditions, including depression. The mechanisms by which exercise and mental health are related are not fully understood. Many medical experts worldwide now acknowledge that exercise has a major impact on a wide range of psychological conditions. It is believed that exercise can be as effective at combating depression as many commonly prescribed drugs.

Now for the good news – there is no need to join a gym. If you want to, then there is certainly no harm in signing up. However, "exercise", in this context, means simple, easy exercises that anybody should be able to manage. Short bursts of activity a few times a day are the type of exercise that experts recommend. A brisk walk lasting only ten minutes is believed to be enough to raise your emotional state for a couple of hours. For those with anxiety disorders, it can be hard to get out and about on occasion. For some, with severe conditions, it can seem impossible. Exercise, however, will help to improve your emotional state and take your mind off anxiety. Use the following tips to increase your chances of successfully incorporating exercise into your life.

Don't start with the intention of completing a 10K run. Use small bursts of activity – the type that gets you a little out of breath and sweating – into the day. Ten minutes every so often is better than half an hour in one go.

Moderate level intensity exercise is recommended as perfect for improving your physical health and also your mental health. That includes walking briskly, cycling, jogging, or swimming. Walking and jogging should not need any investment, and if you're uncomfortable alone, partner up with a friend or relative. Ideally, buddy up with someone who addresses the same issues or has a good understanding of them for extra support.

Psychologists recommend that the exercises you choose should be rhythmic and repetitive. That helps to clear the mind and focus it on the task at hand. Walking, again, is the simplest of these and should be easy to achieve for many people.

If you find that you begin to experience anxiety during a period of exercise, focus your mind on your breathing. Use a meditation technique like "mindfulness meditation" (described briefly in the next chapter) to become aware of your body, breathing simply, and limiting the impact of negative or nervous thoughts. Experience the moment that you are in, not the fears that are in your mind. Alternatively, count each step (out-loud if necessary) to distract your mind from the feelings of anxiety.

Talk About Your Problems with Other People

It helps if you have a trusted friend or relative who is willing to listen to your worries. Trying to contain your feelings can be very challenging. It will just allow your panic to snowball. When a person is willing to listen to your problems and vulnerabilities, you will be a bit more at ease and realize that you are not alone, and secondly, things aren't as bad as they seem.

Do not always expect that the other person will be able to comfort you completely. It is highly unlikely that the other person will be able to erase all your worries. However, talking about worries will prevent them from becoming bigger and bigger. It will prevent you from snapping in an unexpected situation. Talking about your problems will prevent you from exploding and may assist you in maintaining perspective.

Work with a Therapist

Don't be afraid of working with a therapist if your stress or anxiety is severely interfering with your quality of life. Holistic help is only taking the edge off the problem. Therapists are experienced individuals who have been trained to understand what you are going through and can provide that unconditional support to prevent you from descending into more serious anxiety disorders, depression, or stress-related disorders.

Having a Little Fun Never Killed Nobody

Laughing is a great relaxation technique and stress reliever. It increases lots of good feelings and serves to discharge tension. One major problem with people prone to anxiety is that they tend to take life so seriously that they appear to be melancholy all the time, and they eventually stop creating fun moments in their life. Fun and play are essential for the brain's proper functioning; it is a technique that stimulates the brain to come up with creative ideas rather than concentrating on little worries and fears. Within the fun and play, you may develop various ways to apply in situations when you are rendered anxious and helpless. Remember that rigidity limits you to a certain scope of ideas that will directly influence your take on the world.

Conclusion

So, all of these put together will give you just a massive number of herbs and foods that should help kill the herpes simplex virus while healing your body. Herpes ailment is a drawn-out corrupting that is acknowledged by herpes simplex virus (HSV). The genital locale, the oral area, the skin, and the butt-driven district are the body's areas influenced by this sullying. This ailment is known for an incredibly drawn-out stretch, and it commonly assaults people causing several tribulations; some are smooth, and some are perilous.

Genital herpes is one of the most by and large saw kinds of herpes simplex sickness. The genital herpes pollution is an explicitly transmitted affliction that results in genital and butt-driven disturbs. There might be wounds that likewise sway the mouth and face. Dr. Sebi was a notable cultivator that restored many individuals experiencing herpes, and different disorders, for example, disease, aids, hypertension, fibroid, diabetes, body torment, illicit drug use, and so forth.

You know now what Dr. Sebi herpes fix is. Dr. Sebi's answer for herpes is constantly appearing on each side of the world. The purpose behind the so fiery widespread is genuinely not a colossal number of dollars spent on pills or worldwide eminence, considering how some huge name is getting a handle on it. It is to reach the hearts of herpes patients in such a case that its adequacy.

All in all, Dr. Sebi's herpes fix is a compelling one with zero symptoms. When you eat well nourishments, your insusceptible framework will have the quality it needs to fend off intruders. Dr. Sebi's herpes cure is a perpetual solution for herpes, which keeps you away from herpes episodes and encourages you from the different reactions that antivirals may give you. Dr. Sebi's herpes cure can work when done appropriately and with the right spices and the best quality items, so ensure you read the book and even investigate different assets to ensure you are prepared to begin the procedure. In any case, there's as yet an opportunity that this treatment won't work for you and could conceivably work for your companion, relative, neighbor, or who else because your body is not quite the same as their body. Your body may respond an alternate way, so if things don't beat that, it's smarter to make an arrangement and counsel your doctor.

I hope you will be able to implement in your life what you have learned in this book!

HAVE YOU LIKED IT?

To provide the best quality cases to customers, **I would love to hear your thoughts and opinions on my book.**

TO DO SO, I WOULD ENCOURAGE YOU TO <u>LEAVE A HONEST REVIEW ON AMAZON</u>.

The best way to do it? Uploading a brief video with you talking about the **#1** thing you liked the most about this book.

Is it too much for you? Not a problem at all! A simple written review is still an amazing thing!

Your comment will ultimately aid me in continually improving my current and future books. I genuinely hope that your experience with my product was positive and memorable!

<u>THANK YOU IN ADVANCE FOR YOUR VALUABLE FEEDBACK</u>. THIS WILL HELP ME A LOT AS A SELF-PUBLISHED AUTHOR.

Made in the USA
Las Vegas, NV
09 September 2023

77277209R00057